Contraception for Adolescent and Young Adult Women

Amy Whitaker • Melissa Gilliam
Editors

Contraception for Adolescent and Young Adult Women

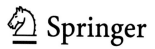 Springer

Editors
Amy Whitaker
Department of Obstetrics
  and Gynecology
Section of Family Planning
  and Contraceptive Research
The University of Chicago
Chicago, IL, USA

Melissa Gilliam
Department of Obstetrics
  and Gynecology
Section of Family Planning
  and Contraceptive Research
The University of Chicago
Chicago, IL, USA

ISBN 978-1-4614-6578-2   ISBN 978-1-4614-6579-9 (eBook)
DOI 10.1007/978-1-4614-6579-9
Springer New York Heidelberg Dordrecht London

Library of Congress Control Number: 2014936413

Printed on acid-free paper

Springer is part of Springer Science+Business Media (www.springer.com)

Preface

Perhaps you are a gynecologist who sees adolescents on an occasional basis, or perhaps you are a pediatrician who provides counseling as your patients reach their teen years, or perhaps you are an expert in adolescent medicine or pediatric gynecology. Regardless, this book was written with you in mind. If you care for adolescents, it will be critical to be knowledgeable about providing and managing contraception as these are among the most commonly prescribed medications for this age group.

In the chapters that follow, you will find contraceptive information written by some of the world's leading experts. They rely on evidenced-based research, new federal guidance, and years of clinical experience in their writing.

The book begins by introducing the topic of contraceptive care for adolescents and the essential elements of the adolescent contraceptive care visit. Clinical pearls for this visit include inquiring about the nature and quality of her relationships, history of sexual assault or abuse, and her sense of well-being within all of her relationships. By the end of the chapter, the reader should be encouraged and understand the personal and public health significance of contraceptive care for adolescents.

The book is subsequently divided into three parts. In the first section, we review each method of contraception. These chapters are written by the leaders in the field of family planning who work closely with these methods as researchers, educators, clinicians, and advocates. Each chapter describes the mechanism of action, side effects, management, and considerations when prescribing the method. The chapters place heavy emphasis on efficacy. While many young women will initiate a contraceptive for medical reasons, it is critical to realize that she may subsequently need the method for contraception. In addition, by reading the chapter on methods available outside of the United States, you may gain insight into products that might one day be available within your practice.

Many of you will work with special populations of young women. The second section of the book will help you take into account special considerations when caring for adolescents who are obese, have medical illness, have disabilities, or are in the postpartum period.

The third section of the book provides guidance as you implement adolescent contraceptive care into your practice. This chapter emphasizes the importance of confidentiality, knowing your local state laws, and being an advocate for the patient at the same time encouraging patient–parent communication. In addition, we treat the topic of sexuality education describing current philosophy as well as the clinician's role as an educator in and out of the clinical setting.

Throughout, this book relies heavily on clinical guidelines particularly the two Centers for Disease Control and Prevention (CDC) publications, the Medical Eligibility Criteria (MEC) and the Selected Practice Recommendations (SPR). The US MEC was created in 2010 and adapted from the rich experience of the World Health Organization in creating evidenced-based recommendations for prescribing contraception specifically with an eye to safety for high-risk women. You will note that there is no method for which age alone is a contraindication. In other words, all contraceptive methods are considered safe for all reproductive age women based on age alone. The SPR is a newer document recently published by the CDC. The SPR provides guidance on contraceptive management: initiation, continuation, and troubleshooting. Thus, these excellent, publically available documents are a cornerstone of this book. Finally, the American Congress of Obstetrics and Gynecology produces clinical guidelines and committee reports that support many of the statements made by the authors.

As adolescents emerge into adulthood, clinicians such as you will be at the forefront of supporting them in achieving their goals for their reproductive health. The majority of adolescents will become sexually active in their teen years. Yet they are likely to use the least effective methods and to use those methods inconsistently and perhaps quitting altogether. Thus, there is a lot of work to be done. This book will help you get started.

Chicago, IL, USA
Amy Whitaker, M.D., M.S.
Melissa Gilliam, M.D., M.P.H.

Contents

Contributors

Romina L. Barral, M.D. Mercy Children's Hospital and Clinics, Kansas City, MO, USA

University of Missouri Kansas City, Kansas City, MO, USA

Adolescent Medicine Division, Department of Pediatrics, Mercy Children's Hospital and Clinics, Kansas City, MO, USA

Deborah Bartz, M.D., M.P.H. Department of Obstetrics, Gynecology, and Reproductive Biology, Brigham and Women's Hospital, Boston, MA, USA

Ellie J. Birtley, B.M., M.F.S.R.H. Solent NHS Trust, Sexual Health, St. Mary's Community Health Campus, Portsmouth, UK

Alison Edelman, M.D., M.P.H. Department of Obstetrics and Gynecology, Oregon Health and Science University, Portland, OR, USA

Eve Espey, M.D., M.P.H. Department of Obstetrics and Gynecology, University of New Mexico, Albuquerque, NM, USA

Melissa Gilliam, M.D., M.P.H. Department of Obstetrics and Gynecology, Section of Family Planning and Contraceptive Research, The University of Chicago, Chicago, IL, USA

Melanie A. Gold, D.O., F.A.A.P. Division of adolescent Medicine, Department of Pediatrics, University of Pittsburgh School of Medicine, Pittsburgh, PA, USA

Cassing Hammond, M.D. Department of Obstetrics and Gynecology, Chicago, IL, USA

Lee Hasselbacher, J.D. Section of Family Planning and Contraceptive Research, Department of Obstetrics and Gynecology, University of Chicago Medicine, Chicago, IL, USA

Elizabeth Janiak, M.A., M.Sc. Department of Obstetrics, Gynecology, and Reproductive Biology, Brigham and Women's Hospital, Boston, MA, USA

Bliss Kaneshiro, M.D., M.P.H. Department of Obstetrics and Gynecology, University of Hawaii, Honolulu, HI, USA

Melissa Kottke, M.D., M.P.H. Department of Gynecology and Obstetrics, Emory University, Atlanta, GA, USA

Patricia A. Lohr, M.D., M.P.H. British Pregnancy Advisory Service, Stratford Upon Avon, UK

Juliana Melo, M.D. Department of Obstetrics and Gynecology, University of Colorado School of Medicine, Aurora, CO, USA

Tanya Pasternack, M.D. Department of Obstetrics and Gynecology, University of New Mexico, Albuquerque, NM, USA

Rachel B. Rapkin, M.D., M.P.H. Department of Obstetrics and Gynecology, University of South Florida, Tampa, FL, USA

Courtney A. Schreiber, M.D., M.P.H. Department of Obstetrics and Gynecology, Hospital of the University of Pennsylvania, Philadelphia, PA, USA

Eleanor Bimla Schwarz, M.D., M.S. Women's Health Services Research Unit, Center for Research on Health Care, University of Pittsburgh, Pittsburgh, PA, USA

Stephanie Sober, M.D. Department of Obstetrics and Gynecology, Hospital of the University of Pennsylvania, Philadelphia, PA, USA

Stephanie Teal, M.D., M.P.H. Department of Obstetrics and Gynecology, University of Colorado School of Medicine, Aurora, CO, USA

Amy Whitaker, M.D., M.S. Department of Obstetrics and Gynecology, Section of Family Planning and Contraceptive Research, The University of Chicago, Chicago, IL, USA

Elisabeth Woodhams, M.D. Department of Obstetrics and Gynecology, Section of Family Planning and Contraceptive Research, The University of Chicago, Chicago, IL, USA

Sloane L. York, M.D., M.P.H. Department of Obstetrics and Gynecology, Rush University Medical Center, Chicago, IL, USA

Mimi Zieman, M.D. SageMed, Atlanta, GA, USA

Chapter 1
Contraceptive Care for Adolescents

Amy Whitaker and Melissa Gilliam

WHY THIS BOOK?

Despite the widespread use of contraception by adolescents, there is no single handbook devoted to the topic. This book is intended to be an easy-to-use clinical guide to contraception for adolescents. This book benefits from the growing expertise in the field of family planning. Indeed, we have assembled some of the world's experts on the topics to write these chapters. Nevertheless, the majority of contraceptive care will take place in busy family planning clinics, board of health clinics, and in offices run by physicians and nurses. The increased research on contraception has not always been coupled with increased communication to practitioners in the field. In addition, a broad array of providers cares for adolescents, including but not limited to pediatricians, internists, family doctors, emergency room doctors, and obstetrician gynecologists. Similarly, many health professionals including doctors, nurses, and health assistants provide frontline care for adolescents. Each of these practitioners needs to be up to date on providing contraceptive care and counseling to adolescent patients. This guide is intended to be a resource for these many areas of specialization. All too often in the absence of information, misinformation arises. Dispelling myths about adolescents and contraception is critical,

A. Whitaker, M.D., M.S. (✉) • M. Gilliam, M.D., M.P.H.
Department of Obstetrics and Gynecology, Section of Family Planning and Contraceptive Research, The University of Chicago,
5841 South Maryland Avenue, MC2050, Chicago, IL 60637, USA
e-mail: awhitaker@babies.bsd.uchicago.edu

A. Whitaker and M. Gilliam (eds.), *Contraception for Adolescent and Young Adult Women*, DOI 10.1007/978-1-4614-6579-9_1,
© Springer Science + Business Media New York 2014

as accurate information will help adolescents adopt the method that works best for them and avoid unwanted pregnancies.

WHY IS IT IMPORTANT?

Of the over six million pregnancies that occur each year in the United States, almost half are unintended (Fig. 1.1). In 2006, 43 % of unintended pregnancies ended in abortion, which was a decrease from 47 % in 2001 [1]. There are important disparities in the rates of unintended pregnancies, with women who are younger, black, poor and those with fewer years of education experiencing the highest rates of unintended pregnancy [1]. Although the general fertility rate has been decreasing in the United States and reached an all-time low in 2011, the proportion of pregnancies that are unintended has remained relatively constant over recent years: 48 % in 1995 and 49 % in 2008 [2, 3]. It is estimated that the direct costs of these unintended pregnancies are $4.6 billion annually. Additionally, up to 53 % of these costs can be attributed to imperfect contraceptive adherence, and one analysis estimates that $288 million dollars per year could be saved if only 10 % of women using oral contraceptive pills (OCPs) switched to more effective long-acting reversible contraceptive (LARC) methods [4]. Public expenditures on family planning and

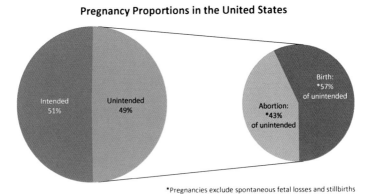

Pregnancy Proportions in the United States

*Pregnancies exclude spontaneous fetal losses and stillbirths

FIG. 1.1 Of the over six million pregnancies that occur each year in the United States, almost half are unintended. (Adapted from Finer 2011).

contraceptive use are extremely cost-effective, with $4 saved for every $1 spent [5].

The majority (89 %) of women at risk for unintended pregnancy use a contraceptive method, and overall use is high among teens 15–19 years old (82 %) and among young adult women 20–24 years (87 %) [2]. However, not all contraception is equal, and almost half of women (48 %) who experience unintended pregnancy report use of a contraceptive method during the month of conception [6].

Given this larger context of the incidence of unintended pregnancy, it is not surprising that the United States has among the highest rates of teen pregnancy of all developed nations. It is over two times higher than that among Canadian and Swedish teens [7]. Over 750,000 teens experience a pregnancy annually, with the highest rates among Hispanic and non-Hispanic black teens. Among all 15–19-year-olds, 82 % of all pregnancies are unintended, and the rate of unintended pregnancy in this age group is 60 per 1,000 women per year. Young adult women aged 20–24 have the highest rate of unintended pregnancy, at 107 per 1,000 annually, with 64 % of all pregnancies in this age group being unintended [1]. The probability that a US woman will experience her first birth by the age of 20 years is 0.18. However, this is strongly influenced by contraceptive use, with a probability of 0.20 for those who used a contraceptive method at first intercourse experiencing first birth by age 20, compared to 0.37 for those who did not (Fig. 1.2a). There are also important racial and ethnic differences, with Latina having the highest probability (0.30) of first birth by the age of 20 compared to non-Hispanic white and non-Hispanic black women (Fig. 1.2b) [8].

The good news is that adolescent pregnancy and adolescent birth rates are decreasing. Teen pregnancy rates declined 42 % from 1990 to 2008, and 2008 was a record low [7]. Despite a slight bump in teen birth from 2005 to 2007, the final 2011 US birth data shows similar decreases in teen birth rates and for women aged 20–24 years, with historic lows in both groups in 2011 [3, 8]. The teen birth rate has dropped by nearly half from 1991 to 2011, from 61.8 to 34.2 per 1,000 women aged 15–19 years. In their report on birth data from 2011, the US Division of Vital Statistics attributes this drop to increased use of contraception as well as public health messaging to teenagers to reduce unintended pregnancy [3]. An in-depth analysis of the decline in teenage pregnancy from 1995 to 2002 showed that increased contraceptive use played a significantly larger

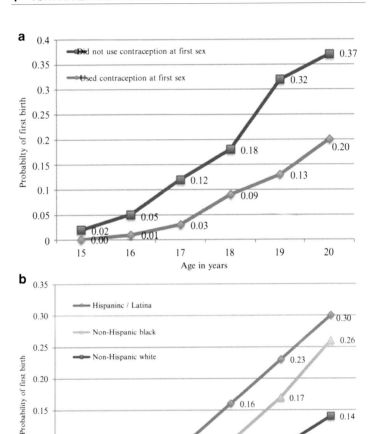

FIG. 1.2 (**a**) Probability of a first birth by age 15, 16, 17, 18, 19, and 20 for females aged 15–24, by use of contraception at first sex: United States 2006–2010. (**b**) Probability of a first birth by age 15, 16, 17, 18, 19, and 20 for females aged 15–24, by Hispanic origin and race: United States 2006–2010. (Adapted from Martinez 2011).

role than the increase in abstinence among teenagers aged 15–19 years (86 % vs. 14 %) [9]. From 1988 to 2006–2010, the use of any contraception at first intercourse increased from 67 to 78 %, use at last intercourse increased from 80 to 86 %, and the use of dual methods of protection (condom plus a hormonal method) increased from 3 to 20 % [8].

While this increase in contraceptive use and dual method use among adolescents over recent years is encouraging, adolescents continue to most commonly use methods with relatively high rates of contraceptive failure and discontinuation. Of sexually active 15–19-year-olds who use any method of contraception, 53 % use oral contraceptive pills (OCPs), 20 % use condoms, 16 % use other hormonal methods, and only 3 % use an intrauterine device (IUD) as their most effective method. Corresponding proportions of 20–24-year-olds are 47 % OCPs, 26 % condoms, 12 % other hormonal, and 6 % IUD (Fig. 1.3) [2]. A recent paper notes that 31 % of women ages 15–24 in a population-based cohort used withdrawal in at least 1 month of the 47-month study period [10].

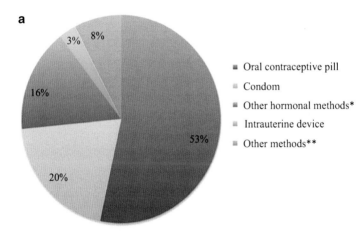

FIG. 1.3 (**a**) Percentage of women aged 15–19 using selected method as their most effective method of contraception (of those who are currently using any method of contraception). (**b**) Percentage of women aged 20–24 using selected method as their most effective method of contraception (of those who are currently using any method of contraception). (**c**), Percentage of women aged 15–44 using selected method as their most effective method of contraception (of those who are currently using any method of contraception). *Other hormonal methods include implantable contraception, injectable contraception, the contraceptive patch, and the contraceptive ring. **Other methods include periodic abstinence and other non-listed methods. (Adapted from Jones 2012).

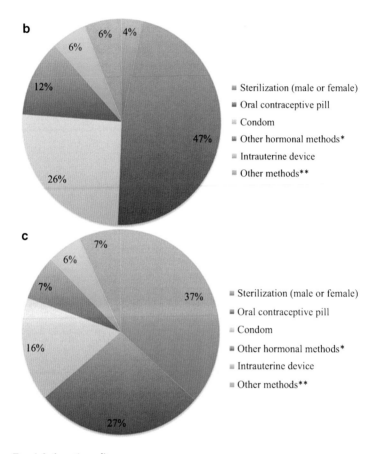

Fɪɢ. 1.3 (continued).

ENCOURAGING THE USE OF LONG-ACTING METHODS

In this book, we discuss all available methods of contraception. However, we have put a special emphasis on the LARC methods, the IUD and the implant. By ordering our chapters roughly from most to least effective methods, we hope to unequivocally convey the message that LARC methods are appropriate for adolescent and young adult women, including nulliparous women. We consider these methods to be highly desirable for use in the adolescent population due to high effectiveness, high rates of continuation, ease of use, and privacy. Because adolescents have a higher rate of discontinuation of shorter acting methods than adult women [11], the long-acting methods may represent a young woman's best option for preventing pregnancy. Some providers are hesitant to use LARC methods, specifically the IUD, for their young and nulliparous patients [12–14], but studies have consistently reported that use among young women is safe, and the American College of Obstetricians and Gynecologists (ACOG) has issued a committee opinion supporting the use of IUDs and implants in adolescent women [15].

While use of LARC increased from 2002 to 2010 for nearly all segments of the population, including teens and young adults, use of LARC among young women is rare [16]. However, this finding does not mean that these methods would not be attractive for the adolescent population if education and access to the methods were more readily available. The Contraceptive CHOICE Project, a longitudinal observational study enrolling over 5,000 women in the St. Louis region that provides no-cost contraception to its participants, attempting to remove cost and access barriers to all methods demonstrated high rates of LARC uptake among adolescents. Like adult women, adolescents aged 14–20 years participating in this trial chose to use LARC methods more frequently than all other methods combined: 70 % of all participants and 62 % of adolescents. Of those who chose a LARC method, the implant was more popular among younger adolescents aged 14–17 years than the IUD (63 % vs. 37 %) while the implant was less likely to be chosen by older adolescents aged 18–20 years (29 % vs. 71 %) [17]. In the 2006–2010 National Survey of Family Growth (NSFG), adolescent and young adult women who reported that they had ever used an IUD were more likely to be parous and report a maternal education of high school or above. Non-Hispanic black women were less likely to report use of an IUD. Use of the implant was too rare in 2010 to perform meaningful analysis of correlates of use among young women [16].

THE ADOLESCENT CLINICAL VISIT

When first meeting an adolescent, it is critical to obtain a detailed history. Often a written intake questionnaire can be helpful for efficiently obtaining substantial information and allowing the patient to provide sensitive information. ACOG provides an excellent adolescent intake form, for both the patient and her parent or guardian, in its Adolescent Took Kit [18]. When using intake forms which request sensitive information, be certain to provide a place for the adolescent to complete the form independent of her parent or guardian. Similarly, it might be best to provide a high-level summary rather than scan these forms so they do not become part of the medical record.

One approach to balance parental involvement with adolescent privacy is to begin the conversation with the parent or guardian present but explain that you would like some time to speak to the adolescent alone, as it helps her to know that she is the patient and can speak to you confidentially. Parents should know that they will not have access to reproductive health records and that adolescents can seek confidential care for sexually transmitted infections (STIs) and contraception (depending on your state laws—see Chap. 13). The parent can be an important part of the early interview: providing medical history, allergies, and family history. However, following this more general conversation, the parent should be asked to leave for all or part of the contraceptive care visit.

When counseling adolescents, asking open-ended questions can build rapport and ensure that the adolescent has an opportunity to discuss what she wants from the visit and can help gauge the adolescent's level of cognitive development. It is important to obtain a full sexual history without judgment or disapproval, including a discussion of oral, anal, or other forms of intercourse that the adolescent may not define as "sex" and therefore may not initially mention. In addition, the clinician should ask about other behaviors such as alcohol, smoking, and drug use which might place the young person at higher risk of poor outcomes.

The goal in contraceptive counseling is to support the adolescent in identifying the method that will work best for her. The conversation should be open and honest without preconceived notions about which method she should choose. Questions such as, "what are you looking for in a contraceptive method?" are open-ended and allow the adolescent to state her needs and desires. Similarly, the clinician should not rule out a method based on age. For example, providers should not assume that an adolescent would not be interested in the IUD, as research has proven this assumption to be incorrect [17]. Clinicians should also identify potential problems or concerns that a patient might have (e.g., missing pills, side effects) and strategize with the patient about what she should do should these occur. Research demonstrates that women are likely to overemphasize risk while underestimating the health benefits of contraceptives. Thus, risks should be discussed with proper perspective, and health benefits should be described [19].

The contraceptive visit is also an ideal time to discuss STIs. Providers can review a variety of risk reduction strategies for STI prevention. These include regular use of condoms, monogamy, avoiding alcohol and drug use, regular STI testing, and use of expedited partner therapy if needed. Adolescents should be instructed in the correct use of a condom. Again, open-ended questions regarding how the adolescent intends to prevent STIs and what barriers she foresees can lead to a productive conversation about adherence. The contraceptive visit may also be a good time to make certain the adolescent has had the human papillomavirus (HPV) vaccine.

Adolescents develop at varying rates; while some are menarcheal at 10, others may just be starting their pubertal development at 13; therefore, careful interviewing and counseling should precede an examination. Oftentimes, there is no need to undress the adolescent for an exam, and remaining clothed may make her more comfortable. In many patients, self-consciousness about their bodies may make the exam difficult to perform. Delaying the genital examination, even with sexually active teens, may prevent them from having reservations about their examiner and allow the rapport to be established more easily. This visit does not necessarily need to include a pelvic examination. Sexually active teens should obtain STI screening annually and with each new sexual partner. With the development of urine and vaginal swab testing for gonorrhea and Chlamydia, STI screening has become easier without the need for a pelvic exam. When a gynecologic exam is indicated, adolescents should be reassured that the examination, while uncomfortable, is not painful.

As in other patients, preventive healthcare should be a part of the examination in this age group. As recommended by ACOG, the initial visit to the obstetrician gynecologist should occur between the ages of 13 and 15 years. During this visit, important components of general health such as immunizations (including the HPV vaccine), risk prevention, and screening for tobacco and substance abuse as well as depression, eating disorders, and obesity should be completed. Screening for cervical cancer via Pap testing is not recommended until age 21 years, regardless of the onset of sexual activity [20].

After the examination, it is helpful to meet again with the family and the patient together. Make a plan together about if and how to discuss reproductive health issues, including contraception, with the parent or guardian before meeting together. Ensure that the adolescent assumes the role of decision-maker and help to empower her to take charge of her own healthcare with her parent or guardian and with your guidance and assistance. Encourage the patient to allow you to be the liaison between her and the family, stressing the benefits of informing everyone of her healthcare needs and the importance of communication, but overall, keep confidentiality consistent with your adolescent patient's needs and desires.

GUIDANCE FROM THE CENTERS
FOR DISEASE CONTROL AND PREVENTION
Throughout this book, we have relied heavily on guidance from the Centers for Disease Control and Prevention (CDC). In 2010, the CDC released the US Medical Eligibility Criteria (MEC) for Contraceptive Use [21]. This document updated contraceptive eligibility criteria with guidance from the World Health Organization MEC, making the criteria more applicable to the US population. Developed using the most recent evidence-based medicine available, the US MEC is an excellent resource to determine if a contraceptive method is appropriate in the context of patients with various characteristics and medical conditions. Many of the chapters refer to the US MEC's categories of medical eligibility for contraceptive use:

1. No restrictions on use
2. Advantages generally outweigh theoretical or proven risks
3. Theoretical or proven risks usually outweigh the advantages
4. Unacceptable health risk

We have included these categories in Appendix A for ease of reference throughout the book. We have also included a summary table of the US MEC in Appendix B. It is important to note that no method of contraception is contraindicated (i.e., receives a category 3 or 4 in the US MEC) based on age alone.

In June of 2013, the CDC released their US Selected Practice Recommendations (US SPR) for Contraceptive Use, which gives specific recommendations for initiating contraceptive methods as well as additional guidance including management of side effects, appropriate screening prior to contraceptive initiation, and follow-up after initiation [22]. Also adapted from the World Health Organization, the US SPR is another excellent resource with evidence-based guidance for providers. When appropriate throughout the book, we have included the US SPR guidance regarding use of specific contraceptive methods. In Appendix C of this book, we have included the US SPR summary table for when to start using contraceptive methods. The US SPR emphasizes that all methods can be started anytime, as long as the provider can be "reasonably certain that the woman is not pregnant." The US SPR suggests that in order to satisfy this condition, a woman must have no signs or symptoms of pregnancy and meet any *one* of the following criteria:

≤7days after start of normal menses, no intercourse since start of last normal menses, correct and consistent use of a reliable method of contraception, ≤7days after spontaneous or induced abortion, and within 4 weeks postpartum, or meet the criteria for lactational amenorrhea (fully or nearly fully breastfeeding, within 6 months postpartum, and amenorrheic) (Appendix C).

ORGANIZATION OF BOOK

The first half of this book is organized by contraceptive method type: IUDs, progestin-only methods, combined hormonal contraception containing both a progestin and estrogen component, barrier methods, as well as emergency contraception. In addition to the basics of the method(s), each chapter includes special attention to the unique aspects of contraceptive care for adolescent patients. As discussed above, recommendations for use and for contraindications to specific methods are consistent with the CDC's evidence-based guidance for contraceptive use. We do not include a chapter on abstinence. Although when used "perfectly," abstinence is 100 % effective at preventing both pregnancy and sexually transmitted infections, we do not consider it appropriate for this clinical guide to contraception. We are writing this book for clinicians to guide them in the care of sexually active or soon-to-be sexually active adolescents, not those young women who have made the choice to remain abstinent. We also do not include a chapter on natural family planning due to its high failure rates and rigorous requirements for correct and consistent use, which make it a less appealing option for the adolescent population.

In the second half of this book, we have assembled expert guidance going beyond the basics of contraceptive use. We include chapters on special populations in which contraceptive decision-making may be difficult for the patient, provider, or both: adolescents with medical illnesses, those with disabilities, obese adolescents, and those in the postpartum period. For these populations, avoiding unintended pregnancy is important as pregnancy has long-lasting and far-reaching health consequences. We have included these chapters separately to give full attention to the challenges and importance of contraception in these populations. Although primarily focused on contraception among adolescents in the United States, we have also included a chapter on emerging methods and those that are not (yet) available in the United States.

Because contraceptive use among adolescents brings up issues extending beyond the clinical environment, we have also included chapters on sexuality education and the legal aspects of minors' access to family planning, with resources to determine state-by-state laws governing contraceptive access by minors. Finally, all methods of contraception fail and nonuse of contraception among young women is common; therefore, we have a chapter on pregnancy option counseling for those adolescents who experience an unintended pregnancy.

SUMMARY

Adolescent pregnancy is decreasing in the United States, but it remains among the highest rates of all developed nations and represents a major public health concern. The decline in adolescent pregnancy is due largely to more and better use of contraceptives. This book will aid clinicians in counseling and encouraging adolescent patients to use effective methods of contraception and ensuring that they are using these methods correctly.

Long-acting contraceptives, implants and IUDs, are highly effective in preventing pregnancy. Use of these methods by adolescents has the potential to significantly decrease the rate of unintended pregnancy in this age group. In this book, we attempt to address some of the common issues that prevent clinicians from recommending these methods. There is no single method of contraception that is right for all women, or for all adolescents. Clinicians must carefully counsel and educate adolescent patients and work with them to find the best method for each individual patient.

REFERENCES

1. Finer LB, Zolna MR. Unintended pregnancy in the United States: incidence and disparities, 2006. Contraception. 2011;84:478–85.
2. Jones J, Mosher W, Daniels K. Current contraceptive use in the United States, 2006–2010, and changes in patterns of use since, 1995. National health statistics reports; no 60. Hyattsville, MD: National Center for Health Statistics; 2012.
3. Martin JA, Hamilton BE, Ventura SJ, Osterman MJK, Mathews TJ. Births: Final data for 2011. National vital statistics reports. Hyattsville, MD: National Center for Health Statistics; 2013. Vol 62 no. 1.
4. Trussell J, Henry N, Hassan F, Prezioso A, Law A, Filonenko A. Burden of unintended pregnancy in the United States: potential savings with increased use of long-acting reversible contraception. Contraception. 2013;87:154–61.
5. Frost JJ, Finer LB, Tapales A. The impact of publicly funded family planning clinic services on unintended pregnancies and government cost savings. J Health Care Poor Underserved. 2008; 19(3):778–96.

6. Finer LB, Henshaw SK. Disparities in rates of unintended pregnancy in the United States, 1994 and 2001. Perspect Sex Reprod Health. 2006;38(2):90–6.
7. Facts on American teen's sexual and reproductive health. Fact Sheet. Guttmacher Institute. 2013.
8. Martinez G, Copen CE, Abma JC. Teenagers in the United States: sexual activity, contraceptive use, and childbearing, 2006–2010 National Survey of Family Growth. Vital Health Stat 23. 2011;31:1–35.
9. Santelli JS, Lindberg LD, Finer LB, Singh S. Explaining recent declines in adolescent pregnancy in the United States: the contribution of abstinence and improved contraceptive use. Am J Public Health. 2007;97:150–6.
10. Dude A, Neustadt A, Martins S, Gilliam M. Use of withdrawal and unintended pregnancy among females 15–24 years of age. Obstet Gynecol. 2013;122:595–600.
11. Rosenstock JR, Peipert JF, Madden T, Zhao Q, Secura GM. Continuation of reversible contraception in teenagers and young women. Obstet Gynecol. 2012;120(6):1298–305.
12. Diaz VA, Hughes N, Dickerson LM, Wessel AM, Carek PJ. Clinician knowledge about use of intrauterine devices in adolescents in South Carolina AHEC. Fam Med. 2011;43:407–11.
13. Kohn JE, Hacker JG, Rousselle MA, Gold M. Knowledge and likelihood to recommend intrauterine devices for adolescents among school-based health center providers. J Adolesc Health. 2012;51:319–24.
14. Tyler CP, Whiteman MK, Zapata LB, Curtis KM, Hillis SD, Marchbanks PA. Health care provider attitudes and practices related to intrauterine devices for nulliparous women. Obstet Gynecol. 2012;119:762–71.
15. Committee on Adolescent Health Care Long-Acting Reversible Contraception Working Group, The American College of Obstetricians and Gynecologists. Adolescents and long-acting reversible contraception: implants and intrauterine devices. Committee Opinion No. 539. Obstet Gynecol. 2012;120:983–8.
16. Whitaker AK, Sisco KM, Tomlinson AN, Dude AM, Martins SL. Use of the intrauterine device among adolescent and young adult women in the United States from 2002 to 2010. J Adolesc Health. 2013;53:401–6.
17. Mestad R, Secura G, Allsworth JE, Madden T, Zhao Q, Peipert JF. Acceptance of long-acting reversible contraceptive methods by adolescent participants in the Contraceptive CHOICE Project. Contraception. 2011;84:493–8.
18. American College of Obstetricians and Gynecologists. Tool kit for teen care; 2nd ed. Washington, DC: ACOG; 2010. http://www.acog.org/About_ACOG/ACOG_Departments/Adolescent_Health_Care/Tool_Kit_for_Teen_Care__Second_EditionTools_for_Adolescent_Assessment [referred to as "ACOG 2010 [1]" in text]. Accessed 11 Nov 2013.

19. Grimes DA, Schulz KF. Nonspecific side effects of oral contraceptives: nocebo or noise? Contraception. 2011;83(1):5–9.
20. Committee opinion no. 460: the initial reproductive health visit. Obstet Gynecol 2010;116:240–3. [referred to as "ACOG 2010 [2]" in text]
21. Centers for Disease Control and Prevention. U.S. medical eligibility criteria for contraceptive use, 2010. MMWR. 2010;59(RR-4):1–86.
22. Centers for Disease Control and Prevention. U.S. selected practice recommendations for contraceptive use, 2013. MMWR Recomm Rep. 2013;62(5):1–64.

Chapter 2
The Intrauterine Device

Eve Espey and Tanya Pasternack

BACKGROUND/EPIDEMIOLOGY OF USE BY TEENS AND YOUNG ADULTS

The intrauterine device (IUD) is an excellent method of contraception for adolescents and young adults. The three IUDs available in the United States include the Copper T380 A and the two levonorgestrel intrauterine systems, one containing 52 mg and one containing 13.5 mg of levonorgestrel. The copper IUD is approved for 10 years of continuous use. The 52 mg levonorgestrel IUD is approved for 5 years and the 13.5 mg for 3 years. IUDs have an outstanding record of safety and effectiveness [1]. Although less research has focused specifically on use of IUDs in teens and young adult women, evidence suggests that the benefits of IUDs—high efficacy, rare complications, and high satisfaction—are similar among younger and older users. The Centers for Disease Control and Prevention (CDC), through the US Medical Eligibility Criteria, supports IUD use in adolescents, indicating that the benefits outweigh the risks [2]. In a Committee Opinion, the American College of Obstetricians and Gynecologists recommend IUDs as first line for nulliparous and parous adolescents [3].

IUDs are underused in the United States, and young women are less likely to use the IUD for contraception than older women. However, IUD use has increased for all groups of women when

E. Espey, M.D., M.P.H. (✉) • T. Pasternack, M.D.
Department of Obstetrics and Gynecology, University of New Mexico,
MSC10 5580, 1, Albuquerque, NM 87131, USA
e-mail: eespey@salud.unm.edu; t_pasternack@yahoo.com

A. Whitaker and M. Gilliam (eds.), *Contraception for Adolescent and Young Adult Women*, DOI 10.1007/978-1-4614-6579-9_2,
© Springer Science + Business Media New York 2014

comparing results from the 2002 to the 2006–2008 National Survey of Family Growth. Although usage rates remain low, women in the under 24 age group had a particularly large increase in long-acting reversible contraceptive (LARC) use [4]. In 2006–2008, 5.6 % of all women used a LARC method; 3.6 % of teens aged 15–19 used such a method (compared to 0.3 % in 2002), and 6.0 % of women aged 20–24 used a LARC method (compared to 1.9 % in 2002) [4].

MECHANISM OF ACTION
The mechanism of action of IUDs is multifactorial. The major effect of the IUD is prevention of fertilization through the creation of a microenvironment toxic to the ovum and sperm [5]. This microenvironment is achieved through the foreign body effect as well as the release of copper ions or levonorgestrel hormone. An inflammatory reaction is created within the uterine cavity that spreads to the genital tract lumen affecting the development and transport of oocytes and spermatozoa. Studies have examined early HCG levels, flushing out the genital tracts of women in early pregnancy and of women with IUDs. They conclude that fertilization does not usually occur in women wearing IUDs. The common belief that the mechanism of action of IUDs is the destruction of an implanted embryo is not supported by evidence. Since the action of IUDs occurs before implantation, the IUD is by definition not an abortifacient.

The levonorgestrel IUDs have additional local and systemic effects. Levonorgestrel is known to increase the viscosity of cervical mucus, obstructing the path of the spermatozoa to the egg. In addition to decreased menstrual flow due to the progesterone effect on the endometrium, about 40 % percent of women have anovulatory cycles due to suppression of FSH and LH [6].

CONTRACEPTIVE EFFICACY AND EFFECTIVENESS
A major advantage of intrauterine contraception is its high effectiveness. Unlike the large gap in effectiveness between perfect and typical use for short-acting contraceptive methods, particularly for adolescents, the gap for IUDs is essentially nonexistent. The proportion of women experiencing an unintended pregnancy within the first year of use of the 52 mg hormonal IUD (levonorgestrel intrauterine system) with both perfect and typical use is 0.2, and for the copper IUD, the proportion is 0.6 for perfect use and 0.8 for typical use [7]. The lower than 1 % failure rate of both IUDs makes them ideal for use in adolescents and young women, a group at high risk for unintended pregnancy.

The Contraceptive CHOICE Project is a large prospective cohort study that has enrolled close to 10,000 women, with the goal of promoting LARC use to decrease unintended pregnancy [8]. Women are counseled about all contraceptive methods, but the effectiveness of LARC methods is emphasized. Additionally, since the project funds all contraceptive methods, study subjects face no financial barriers to obtaining their method of choice. With this approach, 75 % of women in the study chose a LARC method. In a recent analysis of 7,486 participants, the superior effectiveness of LARC methods in preventing unintended pregnancy was clearly demonstrated. Contraceptive failure with pills, patch, and ring users was 4.55 per 100 participant-years vs. 0.27 among LARC users. In other words, the risk of failure with pills, patch, and ring was 20 times higher than with LARC methods. This analysis also emphasized the lower effectiveness of short-acting methods in teens. In women under age 21 using pills, patch, or ring, the risk of unintended pregnancy was almost twice as high as that of older women. The proportion of teens experiencing an unintended pregnancy with the IUD was <1 %; there was no difference in effectiveness of the IUD based on age.

SIDE EFFECTS

The major side effects of both the copper and the hormone IUD include bleeding and pain. In a large Brazilian study, adolescents had a higher rate of copper IUD removal than parous adults, mostly due to problems with pain and bleeding [9]. In a prospective cohort study of teens who chose an IUD for contraception, bleeding and pain were the two major side effects for which teens requested removal [10], but the rate of discontinuation of both devices was similar, as was the time frame of request for removal. Additionally, removal requests were not clustered within a few months of insertion.

Women using the levonorgestrel IUD rarely complain of hormone side effects because the dose of hormone released by the IUD is small and mostly acts locally within the endometrium. In the Contraceptive Choice study, 3 % of women using a levonorgestrel IUD discontinued use due to perceived side effects of acne and weight change [11].

Satisfaction and continuation are often a proxy for the severity of side effects of a contraceptive method. Continuation rates for IUDs in adolescents and young women are high. Similarly, satisfaction rates appear high in the limited number of prospective studies addressing adolescents and young women. Retrospective studies, including a small case series of Canadian teens and a small study of New Zealand teens using the levonorgestrel IUD, show high satisfaction [12, 13]. In a trial with a large number of adolescents, over 84 % of participants were somewhat or very satisfied with IUDs compared to 53 % using non-long-acting methods [11].

CONTINUATION

Continuation rates for IUDs are generally high in adolescents and young adults. Two recent studies examined continuation rates in young women: In the Contraceptive Choice study, 12-month continuation for the 52 mg levonorgestrel IUD was similar to that of older adults at 88 %, but continuation for the copper IUD was 72 % for adolescents compared with 85 % for older women [11]. Satisfaction rates for both IUDs were high. In a recent study of parous adolescents, 12-month continuation was 55 % for both copper and levonorgestrel IUDs [10]. Even at the lower end of the range, continuation rates of around 50 % are higher than those for short-acting methods. Continuation rates for teens for the patch, DMPA, ring, and pills ranged from 10.9 per 100 person-years to 32.7 per 100 person-years [14] and were the lowest for the patch and DMPA. Higher rates of discontinuation of all shorter-acting methods were associated with younger age. Reasons for discontinuation of IUDs include expulsion, request for removal for bleeding and pain, and desire for pregnancy.

In a small, randomized controlled trial, 23 teens aged 14–18 desiring an IUD for contraception were assigned either to a levonorgestrel IUD or to the Copper T380 A IUD [15]. At 6-month follow-up, 75 % of the hormone IUD group and 45 % of the copper IUD group were still using the IUD. The difference was not significantly different, given the small sample size. Two partial expulsions occurred in the copper IUD group. Satisfaction in those continuing the IUD was high in both groups.

Studies conflict about a higher risk of expulsion associated with young age and/or nulliparity [10, 16]. In a cohort study of adolescent mothers who received an IUD for contraception, higher than expected rates of expulsion occurred: 13.3 % for the levonorgestrel IUD and 16.7 % for the copper IUD [10]. These results, however, should be interpreted with caution in light of the CHOICE study, with its finding of significantly lower risk of unintended pregnancy in adolescent women using LARC methods. Request for removal for bleeding and pain appears similar between younger and older IUD users [10, 16]. Overall, among teens and young women, long-acting methods such as the IUD and implant are associated with less unintended pregnancy and repeat pregnancy than with shorter-acting methods [17, 18].

CONTRAINDICATIONS

Since there are few contraindications to IUD use, almost all women are eligible for intrauterine contraception. The World Health Organization (WHO) and CDC have developed evidence-based medical eligibility criteria for contraceptive use (US MEC) [2, 19]. Guidelines are assigned a rating of one through four based on risk (Appendix A); in some cases there are separate recommendations for initiation and continuation of use. Contraindications most likely to affect adolescents and young women are pregnancy, anatomic abnormalities, active PID, and active sexually transmitted infections (STIs). Anatomic abnormalities are relatively common in young women and include Mullerian anomalies such as septa or uterus didelphys. Although scant data exist about IUD use in the setting of uterine anomalies, it may be useful to consider insertion on a case-by-case basis, depending on the particular anomaly [20]. It is important to note that while current PID and current STIs are given a US MEC Category 4 (condition represents an unacceptable health risk) rating for initiation of an IUD, both are given a Category 2 rating for continuation of an IUD. Providers may jump to removal of an IUD, particularly in a younger woman, in the setting of cervicitis or PID, whereas it may be acceptable to retain the IUD, treat the infection with appropriate antibiotics, and recommend close follow-up with reassessment in 48–72 h to verify clinical and microbiologic resolution of the infection [21]. The clinical course of PID does not appear to change based on whether or not the IUD is retained or removed [2]. (See Appendix B for summary of US MEC, including recommendations regarding IUDs).

TIMING OF INSERTION AND FOLLOW-UP

Although some sources recommend inserting an IUD during menses, the US SPR states that an IUD can be inserted anytime the provider can be reasonably certain that a woman is not pregnant. Additional contraception (or abstinence) is recommended for 7 days if a levonorgestrel IUD is inserted >7 days after the first day of menses, but no additional contraception is required for the copper IUD regardless of timing of insertion [21] (see Appendix C).

It is unclear whether follow-up after IUD insertion is necessary, but a "string check," usually scheduled 3–4weeks after IUD insertion is customary. At this check, a speculum exam and bimanual exam are performed to identify the strings and to rule out partial expulsion, which may occur more frequently than complete expulsion. Additionally, the bimanual exam may identify signs of systemic infection.

The US Selected Practice Recommendations for Contraceptive Use recommend having a woman return to discuss side effects, if she wants to change her method, and when it is time to remove or replace the IUD. The recommendations state that no routine follow-up visit is required; however, some populations, including adolescents may benefit from more frequent follow-up visits [21].

ISSUES FOR ADOLESCENTS AND YOUNG WOMEN
Lack of Familiarity with IUDs

A major issue for adolescents and young women is unfamiliarity with IUDs and their advantages. Several studies corroborate young women's lack of knowledge about the method [22–24]. In a questionnaire of young women seeking emergency contraception, over half reported they did not know whether the IUD was more or less effective or had` more or fewer side effects than the pill [24]. In a survey of teens attending a family planning clinic, only 19 % had heard of an IUD [23]. In a study of young pregnant women aged 14–25, only half had heard of an IUD and those who had heard of it were more likely to be older and parous [22].

Restrictive Criteria Excluding Teens and Nulliparous Women from IUD Use

Many providers use restrictive criteria to define an appropriate candidate for IUDs, further limiting young women's access both to knowledge about and use of the method. In a survey of physicians, nurse practitioners, and physician assistants, knowledge gaps about IUDs were common, and only 39 and 45 % of respondents respectively, would offer an IUD to a teenager or to a nulliparous woman [25].

Many adolescent and young women are nulliparous; some providers have specific concerns about the use of IUDs in nulliparous women, namely concerns about infection, pain with insertion, and increased side effects. The 52 mg levonorgestrel IUD remains off-label for use in nulliparous women although a growing body of evidence demonstrates safety and efficacy in nulliparous women [26] and the US MEC gives a Category 2 rating for use of both the copper and hormone IUDs in nulliparous women. As with parous women, nulliparous women have higher satisfaction rates with IUDs than with short-acting methods [2]. No studies show higher rates of PID or infertility in nulliparous women [27]. A large case–control study examining risk factors for tubal infertility did not show an increased risk of PID in women who had been IUD users but rather in women with a positive chlamydia antibody, demonstrating that STIs, not IUDs, are likely responsible for PID that may lead to infertility [27]. Pain with insertion may be greater for nulliparous women, but evidence is reassuring that overall pain scores for IUD insertion are low for both nulliparous and parous women [28].

Rapid Repeat Pregnancy

Teens are at high risk for rapid repeat pregnancy, defined as a second pregnancy within 24 months of delivery. The negative consequences of bearing multiple children in adolescence include lack of educational attainment and poverty. Approximately 20–66 % of teen mothers experience repeat pregnancy within a year of delivery [29]; minority adolescent women have higher rates of rapid repeat pregnancy than whites. The postpartum time period is critical for initiating contraception to prevent rapid repeat pregnancy.

Postpartum IUD Initiation in Teens

A qualitative study of 20 postpartum African American teens desiring an IUD examined factors that prevented, delayed, or supported their ability to receive it [30]. Barriers included providers' restrictive criteria for candidate selection, lack of insurance coverage, fear of side effects, and delay in placement. An important facilitative factor was a strong positive message from providers promoting IUD use.

The most promising strategy for reducing rapid repeat pregnancy in teens is the use of LARC methods [17]. In a recent prospective cohort study of pregnant adolescents, 65 % intended to use a LARC method [31], confirming the high uptake seen in the CHOICE study, given appropriate counseling. Of the 65 % who desired LARC for postpartum contraception, only 63 % actually received it, and implant intenders were more likely to receive the method than IUD intenders. In this study setting, the implant was placed prior to hospital discharge, whereas the IUD was placed at the traditional 6-week postpartum visit. Notably, over half of the adolescents intending the IUD resumed intercourse prior to receiving their contraceptive method. The study suggests that optimal timing for initiation of LARC methods is immediately postpartum.

CONCLUSION

Although studies specific to IUD use in adolescents are urgently needed, existing evidence is reassuring that adolescents are excellent candidates for the IUD. Teens experience unique challenges in preventing unintended pregnancy and rapid repeat pregnancy and are much more likely to experience contraceptive failure using short-acting methods than older women. IUDs hold a number of advantages for adolescents, including ease of use, effectiveness, and rapid reversibility. IUDs should be considered a first-line choice for all women, including adolescents [16].

REFERENCES

1. American College of Obstetricians and Gynecologists. ACOG Practice Bulletin No. 121: long-acting reversible contraception: implants and intrauterine devices. Obstet Gynecol. 2011;118(1):184–96.
2. Centers for Disease Control and Prevention (CDC). U.S. Medical Eligibility Criteria for Contraceptive Use, 2010. MMWR Recomm Rep. 2010;59(RR–4):1–86.
3. American College of Obstetricians and Gynecologists. Adolescents and long-acting reversible contraception: implants and intrauterine devices. Committee Opinion No. 539. Obstet Gynecol. 2012;120:983–8.
4. Kavanaugh ML, Jerman J, Hubacher D, Kost K, Finer L. Characteristics of women in the United States who use long-acting reversible contraceptive methods. Obstet Gynecol. 2011;117:1349–57.
5. Ortiz ME, Croxatto H. Copper-T intrauterine device and levonorgestrel intrauterine system: biological bases of their mechanism of action. Contraception. 2007;75(6 Suppl):S16–31.
6. Rivera R, Yacobson I, Grimes D. The mechanism of action of hormonal contraceptives and intrauterine contraceptive devices. Am J Obstet Gynecol. 1999;181:1263–9.
7. Trussell J. Contraceptive failure in the United States. Contraception. 2011;83:397–404.
8. Winner B, Peipert J, Zhao Q, Buckel C, Madden T, Allsworth J, Secura G. Effectiveness of long-acting reversible contraception. N Engl J Med. 2012;366(21):1998–2007.
9. Diaz J, Pinto A, Bahamondes L, et al. Performance of the copper T200 in parous adolescents: are copper IUDs suitable for these women? Contraception. 1993;48:23–8.
10. Teal SB, Sheeder J. IUD use in adolescent mothers: retention, failure and reasons for discontinuation. Contraception. 2012;85:270–4.
11. Peipert JF, Zhao Q, Allworth JE, Petrosky E, Madden T, Eisenberg D, et al. Continuation and satisfaction of reversible contraception. Obstet Gynecol. 2011;117:1105–13.
12. Toma A, Jamieson MA. Revisiting the intrauterine contraceptive device in adolescents. J Pediatr Adolesc Gynecol. 2006;19:291–6.
13. Paterson H, Ashton J, Harrison-Woolrych M. A nationwide cohort study of the use of the levonorgestrel intrauterine device in New Zealand adolescents. Contraception. 2009;59:433–8.
14. Raine TR, Foster-Rosales A, Upadhyay UD, Boyer CB, Brown BA, Sokoloff A, Harper CC. One-year contraceptive continuation and pregnancy in adolescent girls and women initiating hormonal contraceptives. Obstet Gynecol. 2011;117:363–71.
15. Godfrey EM, Memmel LM, Neustadt A, Shah M, Nicosia A, Moorthie M, Gilliam M. Intrauterine contraception for adolescents aged 14-18years: a multicenter randomized pilot study of levonorgestrel-releasing intrauterine system compared to the Copper T-380 A. Contraception. 2010;81:123–7.

16. Deans EI, Grimes DA. Intrauterine devices for adolescents: a systematic review. Contraception. 2009;79:418–22.
17. Stevens-Simon C, Kelly L, Kulick R. A village would be nice but… it takes a long-acting contraceptive to prevent repeat adolescent pregnancies. Am J Prev Med. 2001;21:60–5.
18. Zibners A, Cromer BA, Hayes J. Comparison of continuation rates for hormonal contraception among adolescents. J Pediatr Adolesc Gynecol. 1999;12:90–4.
19. World Health Organization. Medical eligibility criteria for contraceptive use. 4th ed. Geneva: WHO; 2009. http://whqlibdoc.who.int/publications/2010. Accessed 5 Mar 2012.
20. Tepper N, Zapata L, Jamieson D, Curtis K. Use of intrauterine devices in women with uterine anatomic abnormalities. Int J Gynaecol Obstet. 2010;109(1):52–4.
21. Centers for Disease Control and Prevention (CDC). U.S. selected practice recommendations for contraceptive use, 2013. MMWR Recomm Rep. 2013;62(5):1–64.
22. Stanwood NL, Bradley KA. Young pregnant women's knowledge of modern intrauterine devices. Obstet Gynecol. 2006;108:1417–22.
23. Whitaker AK, Johnson LM, Harwood B, Chiappetta L, Creinin MD, Gold MA. Adolescent and young adult women's knowledge of and attitudes toward the intrauterine device. Contraception. 2008;78:211–7.
24. Schwarz EB, Kavanaugh M, Douglas E, Dubowitz T, Creinin MD. Interest in intrauterine contraception among seekers of emergency contraception and pregnancy testing. Obstet Gynecol. 2009;113:833–9.
25. Harper CC, Blum M, de Thiel Bocanegra H, Darney PD, Speidel JJ, Policar M, et al. Challenges in translating evidence to practice. Obstet Gynecol. 2008;111:1359–69.
26. Use of the Mirena LNG-IUS and Paragard CuT380A intrauterine devices in nulliparous women. Society of Family Planning Guideline #20092. Posted with permission of Elsevier, Inc. Originally published in Contraception 81:5(2010), pp. 367–371.
27. Hubacher D, Lara-Ricalde R, Taylor DJ, Guerra-Infante F, Guzman-Rodriguez R. Use of copper intrauterine devices and the risk of tubal infertility among nulligravid women. N Engl J Med. 2001;345:561–7.
28. Hubacher D, Reyes V, Lillo S, Zepeda A, Chen PL, Croxatto H. Pain from copper intrauterine device insertion: randomized trial of prophylactic ibuprofen. Am J Obstet Gynecol. 2006;195:1272–7.
29. Raneri LG, Wiemann CM. Social ecological predictors of repeat adolescent pregnancy. Perspect Sex Reprod Health. 2007;39:39–47.
30. Weston M, Martins S, Neustadt A, Gilliam M. Factors influencing uptake of intrauterine devices among postpartum adolescents: a qualitative study. Am J Obstet Gynecol. 2012;206:40. e1–7.
31. Tocce K, Sheeder J, Python J, Teal SB. Long acting reversible contraception in postpartum adolescents: Early initiation of etonogestrel implant is superior to IUDs in the outpatient setting. J Pediatr Adolesc Gynecol. 2012;25:59–63.

Chapter 3
Progestin-Only Contraception

Romina L. Barral and Melanie A. Gold

BACKGROUND

Progestin-only contraceptives (POCs) play an important role in contraceptive management. They present advantages over combined hormonal contraception (CHC) in women with contraindications to estrogens. Progestins, when given alone, carry very few cardiovascular risks and most progestins used in contraception do not adversely affect clotting factors. Conversely, adolescents with medical conditions may benefit from POCs. Overall studies of women with sickle cell disease suggest it may be particularly beneficial to use depot medroxy progesterone acetate (DMPA) because of a reduction in sickle crises; the Centers for Disease Control and Prevention Medical Eligibility Criteria (US MEC) has recommended that sickle cell anemia be classified as a Category 1 for POCs (a condition for which there is no contraindication for the use of the method; see Appendix A) [1]. In addition, POCs do not cause estrogen-related effects such as nausea, edema and

R.L. Barral, M.D. (✉)
Mercy Children's Hospital and Clinics, Kansas City, MO, USA

University of Missouri Kansas City, Kansas City, MO, USA

Adolescent Medicine Division, Department of Pediatrics,
Mercy Children's Hospital and Clinics, Kansas City, MO, USA
e-mail: rlbarral@cmh.edu

M.A. Gold, D.O., F.A.A.P.
Division of adolescent Medicine, Department of Pediatrics,
University of Pittsburgh School of Medicine, Pittsburgh, PA, USA
e-mail: magold@pitt.edu

A. Whitaker and M. Gilliam (eds.), *Contraception for Adolescent and Young Adult Women*, DOI 10.1007/978-1-4614-6579-9_3,

breast tenderness. Finally, if a woman is hesitant to use exogenous estrogens, she may feel more comfortable using POCs instead. Of note, in contrast to combination methods, POCs have not been proven to consistently improve acne, suppress ovarian cyst formation, prevent ovarian cancer or give predictable menstrual control. In summary, POCs offer a safe alternative to combination methods, with particular benefits and without the adverse effects or health risks associated with estrogens [2].

POCs have been available for routine contraception since the 1960s, and several new progestins have been synthesized for use in contraceptives over the past five decades. The most potent progestins can be used at very low doses and be delivered via oral or non-oral long-acting delivery systems. Three main formulations available in the United States include progestin-only pills (POPs), DMPA, and etonogestrel implants.

CHARACTERISTICS BY METHOD
Progestin-Only Pills
The progestin dose is lower in POPs compared to the dose in combination oral contraceptives (hence being called the "mini-pill"). Worldwide, commercially available POPs contain low doses of levonorgestrel, norethindrone (norethisterone), ethynodiol diacetate, or desogestrel. In the United States, the only available POPs contain 0.35 mg norethindrone (Micronor®, Nor-QD®, Jolivette®, Camila®, Heather®, Nora-BE® or Errin®). Packs of POPs contain 28 active pills (there are no placebo pills or hormone free-week) and, for maximum efficacy, must be taken within 3 h of the same time every day. POPs thicken cervical mucus making it relatively impenetrable to sperm; they alter ciliary action in the fallopian tubes, and thin the lining of the endometrium making implantation unlikely. Inhibition of ovulation is variable with POPs and is not the primary mechanism of action. The first POPs introduced in the early 1970s (containing levonorgestrel 30 mg or norethisterone 300 mg) variably inhibited ovulation, leading to lower contraceptive efficacy compared to combination oral contraceptive pills (COCs) when consistently and correctly used (0.5 pregnancies per 100 woman-years for POPs compared to 0.1 per 100 woman-years for COC pills). In contrast, POPs containing desogestrel 75 mg prevent 99 % of ovulations. Unfortunately, no POPs containing desogestrel are available in the United States [3, 4].

Ideally, POPs are intiated during the first 5 days of the menstrual period but may be started any time it can be reasonably certain that the woman is not pregnant (see Appendix C). If POPs are started outside of this window, women should use a back up method such as a condom (or abstain from sexual intercourse) for 2 days [5, 6]. They can also be initiated right after switching from another method (the day after stopping another hormonal method, with no breaks in between), immediately post-partum (please see details in post-partum Chap. 11), or immediately after abortion or miscarriage [5]. If switching from COCs, the contraceptive ring or patch, a woman should skip the placebo week, and start POPs right after the last day of active combination pill or last day of ring or patch use. The change in cervical mucus induced by POPs requires 2–4 h to occur. Mucus impermeability diminishes after 22 h with some sperm penetration occurring by 24 h. If a POP dose is missed, i.e., is taken after the 3-h window period, one POP should be taken as soon as possible. The woman should continue taking the pill daily at the same time each day, even if it means taking two pills on the same day, and abstain from sexual intercourse or use a back-up method for 2 days. Emergency contraception should be considered if the woman has had unprotected intercourse [5]. Women who discontinue POPs have an immediate return of fertility, regardless of the duration of use since POPs do not reliably inhibit ovulation and cervical mucus thins 24 h after the last POP is taken. Caution should be used when taking rifampicin, certain anticonvulsants and anti-retrovirals, as well as St. John's wort. These medications have been shown to have less interaction with POPs compared to COCs. Regardless, a back up contraceptive method such as a condom is recommended when taking any of these medications and POPs simultaneously.

The pill-taking regimen for POPs is fixed: the same color pill is taken every day at the same time without a "placebo" week; there are no days without pill-taking and there are no placebo pills in the pack. Since POPs do not contain estrogen, there is no increase in risk of stroke, myocardial infarction and venous thromboembolism [7]. COCs, contraceptive rings, and patches can cause nausea, vomiting, breast tenderness, mood changes, and bloating; all symptoms that frequently cause young women to discontinue treatment. POPs may be a good choice when an adolescent wants an oral contraceptive but cannot tolerate estrogen-related side effects. Hormone-dependent headache (on the active pills) and menstrual migraine (which often occur on the inactive pills) are two common adverse effects reported with COC use. POPs may also be a good choice in these clinical situations because there are no hormone free days and the dose of progestin is so low that it is less likely to provoke hormonally induced headaches. In conclusion, POPs are an effective form of estrogen-free contraception that may be appealing to adolescents for whom estrogens are contraindicated. Due to the limited duration of action compared to COCs, adherence to POPs may be particularly difficult yet they may be an acceptable alternative that should be offered to adolescents who want an oral progestin-only contraceptive method.

Depot Medroxyprogesterone Acetate

DMPA is the only injectable contraceptive currently available in the United States; it was approved by the Food and Drug Administration (FDA) for contraceptive use in October 1992. Its intramuscular (IM) formulation consists of 150 mg of medroxy-progesterone acetate (a pregnane 17α-hydroxyprogesterone deriv-ative) in an aqueous suspension of microcrystals in a lipid base, and is administered in the gluteal or deltoid area every 13 weeks. This preparation works as a long-acting delivery system due to the low solubility of the microcrystals. The FDA approved a micronized formulation of 104 mg DMPA in December 2004 to be administered subcutaneously in either the abdomen or thigh (DMPA-SC). The option of self-administration is particularly attractive since the need to attend an office visit every 12 weeks for an injection is a barrier, especially for adolescent women, and a possible reason for adolescents stopping the method or getting late injections. Despite the potential appeal of self-administration, to date the manufacturer has not developed and marketed an auto-injector for use by women at home.

DMPA inhibits follicular development and ovulation. The pro-gestin's negative feedback on the hypothalamus inhibits the pulse frequency of gonadotropin-releasing hormone (GnRH), which decreases the release of follicle-stimulating hormone (FSH) and luteinizing hormone (LH) by the anterior pituitary. Decreased lev-els of FSH inhibit follicular development, preventing an increase in estradiol levels. This negative feedback and lack of estrogen positive feedback on LH release prevents the LH surge which prevents ovulation. DMPA also thickens cervical mucus and thins the endometrial lining. Some literature also suggests alteration of tubal motility [8].

DMPA may be initiated anytime, if the patient and provider can be reasonably certain that the patient is not pregnant (see Appendix C). If it has been >7 days since the first day of the patient's last menstrual cycle, she should use a back-up method (or abstain from sexual intercourse) for 7 days [5]. However if the patient is pregnant at time of injection, no teratogenic or other adverse effects on the pregnancy have been shown [9, 10]. Thus, if a provider cannot be certain that a patient is not pregnant, it is reasonable to give the DMPA injection, with a follow-up pregnancy test in 2–4 weeks [5]. If unprotected intercourse occurs within the first 7 days post-injection, emergency contraception should be offered. When switching from another contraceptive method to DMPA, the injection should be given in a manner that ensures continuation of contraceptive coverage, which may include extending use of the previous method (including other hormonal methods or an IUD) 7 days after the first DMPA injection [5]. There is an effective grace period of 2 weeks that allows for late injections (thus, up to 15 weeks after the last injection) without the use of a back-up method of contraception [5]. If an adolescent returns for reinjection *after* 15 weeks, she may have the injection if the provider can be reasonably sure that she is not pregnant, and she should use a back up method of contraception (or abstain from intercourse) for 7 days [5]. The option of emergency contraception should be considered if appropriate. There are no time limits on shortening the interval between injections, so a repeat DMPA injection can be given early when necessary [5].

DMPA can be used while breastfeeding, the concentration of the drug is negligible in breast milk and no adverse effects on infant growth or development have been observed. While the efficacy of both the IM and SC formulations of DMPA decreases after 14–16 weeks from the last injection, women should be counseled that ovulation can take up to 10 months to return. DMPA is a particularly good contraceptive choice for adolescents who are taking cytochrome P450 inducers for treatment of mood disorders, seizure disorders, migraine, etc., since they cause minimal drug interactions with DMPA (compared to POPs, COCs, and implants). Aminoglutethimide, a treatment for Cushing's syndrome, when administered concomitantly with DMPA may significantly depress the serum concentrations of medroxyprogesterone acetate.

DMPA offers a number of potential benefits to adolescents. It does not require a daily action, is highly effective, and provides a grace period for delayed injection. In addition, DMPA is private, is not coital dependent, and does not require partner involvement. For young women with sickle cell disease, DMPA is particularly beneficial because it reduces the incidence of sickle cell crises [11]. Likewise, for women with seizure disorders, DMPA raises the seizure threshold resulting in fewer seizure episodes [12, 13]. Amenorrhea is seen with long-term use (50 % after the first year of use, 75 % after 2 years and 80 % by 5 years of use) [6]. This side effect is frequently desired by teens. Other benefits include decreased incidence of iron deficiency anemia, primary dysmenorrhea, endometriosis, ovulation pain, and functional ovarian cysts. DMPA also decreases risk of endometrial cancer by 80 % and decreases the incidence of uterine fibroids and ectopic pregnancies. Because DMPA creates thick mucus and amenorrhea, there is a decreased incidence of PID in adolescents with cervicitis who use DMPA. For these reasons, DMPA has become a popular contraceptive choice and is widely used among adolescents and young adults in the United States. Approximately 9.4 % of all female adolescents, aged 15–19 years, use DMPA as their contraceptive method ([14]; NSFG 2006–2008 cycle).

Implants

Nexplanon®, formerly marketed as Implanon®, manufactured by Merck & Co., is the only implant currently marketed in the United States. It consists of a 40 mm × 2 mm single rod containing 68 mg of etonogestrel (ENG), the biologically active metabolite of desogestrel, covered with a rate-controlling membrane of ethylene vinyl acetate that slowly releases the hormone. The FDA approved the ENG implant in July 2006. Several studies have confirmed its high efficacy, convenience, and cost-effectiveness, however, restricted availability of trained providers, limited marketing, and initial cost contribute to its limited use in the United States. Proper subdermal implant insertion facilitates removal. Studies show both insertion and removal can be completed in a few minutes as an outpatient procedure by a trained clinician (insertion mean time: 0.5 min; 3.5 min for removal; [15]). Nexplanon® prescribing information recommends subdermal insertion approximately 8–10 cm (3–4 in.) above the medial epicondyle of the humerus, in the inner aspect of the non-dominant arm (Figs. 3.1 and 3.2). The device maintains contraceptive efficacy for 3 years. The ENG implant suppresses ovulation, thickens cervical mucus, and thins the endometrial lining. Implant labeling data indicates pregnancies could occur as early as 7–14 days after removal. Therefore, another form of contraception should be started immediately after removal of the implant to provide continued contraceptive protection. Certain anticonvulsants and anti-retrovirals as well as Rifampicin can decrease the effectiveness of the implant.

The implant can be inserted any time if it is reasonably certain that the woman is not pregnant (see Appendix C). If it is inserted after day 5 of the menstrual cycle, she needs to use a back-up method of contraception or abstain from sexual intercourse for 7 days. If switching from another method and not within 5 days of the start of the last menses, that method may be continued for an additional 7 days after insertion of the implant [5]. The implant package instructions advises inserting the implant within 5 days

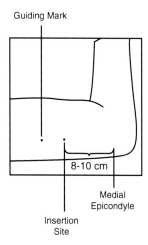

Guiding Mark

8-10 cm

Medial
Epicondyle

Insertion
Site

FIG. 3.1 Anatomic references for insertion. Adapted from Nexplanon prescribing information. Reproduced with permission of Merck Sharp & Dohme B.V., a subsidiary of Merck & Co., Inc., Whitehouse Station, New Jersey, USA. All rights reserved.

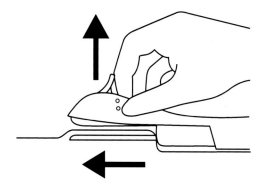

FIG. 3.2 Insertion. Adapted from Nexplanon prescribing information. Reproduced with permission of Merck Sharp & Dohme B.V., a subsidiary of Merck & Co., Inc., Whitehouse Station, New Jersey, USA. All rights reserved.

following a first trimester abortion and on days 21–28 following a second trimester abortion. However, the US MEC assigns a category one for post-abortion placement in both the first and second trimesters, as well as immediately after septic abortion, and the US SPR states that the implant may be inserted immediately after spontaneous or induced abortion without reference to gestational age at the time of abortion. For post-partum women who are not breastfeeding the implant can be inserted immediately after delivery. For women who are post-partum and breast-feeding, the implant can also be inserted at any time (US MEC Category 2 for <1 month postpartum and US MEC category 1 if ≥1 month postpartum), if it is reasonably certain that the woman is not pregnant [5]. The use of the ETG-releasing implant in the immediate postpartum period was not associated with deleterious maternal clinical or metabolic effects or effects on newborn growth. In addition, users of the ETG-releasing implant showed greater reductions in body mass index (BMI) (kg/m^2) and weight within 6 weeks after delivery [16].

ENG implants provide highly effective, discreet, easy to use, convenient, long acting estrogen-free contraception, making it an ideal choice for adolescents. It also represents a good choice for postpartum women whose risk for a blood clot is elevated and for whom estrogen are contraindicated. A prospective study of contraceptive choices in teenage mothers recruited from the adolescent antenatal service or who delivered within 5 days postpartum at King Edward Memorial Hospital of Western Australia highlighted the advantages of the ENG implant over other contraceptive methods for this population. The implant was an acceptable and effective method for reducing repeat pregnancy within 24-months postpartum and teens using the implant had a higher rate of continuation at 24-months postpartum when compared with COC and DMPA using teens ($p < 0.001$). The mean duration for implant use was 18.7 months (95 % CI, 17.0–20.3) compared to 11.9 months (95 % CI, 9.5–14.3) for COC/DMPA use. In a self-administered questionnaire, 137 girls younger than 18 years old reported liking that they did not have to remember to use the implant, that it was long lasting, and that it was effective and convenient. This study also suggested that waiting until 6 weeks post-partum to insert the implant might be too late (adolescents were already sexually active by then) and, therefore if an adolescent mother is agreeable to contraception, the implant should be inserted before postnatal discharge and use should be reinforced at a 4- to 6-week postnatal appointment [17]. The ENG implant effectively inhibits ovulation by preventing LH surge and inhibits endometrial proliferation. These two effects explain its use as an option in the hormonal treatment of endometriosis [18]. Funk et al. reported an 81 % improvement in dysmenorrhea among 18- to 40-year-old women who used the ENG implant and presented with a baseline history of dysmenorrhea. Differences in bleeding patterns during

ENG implant use were not correlated with reported incidence or severity of dysmenorrhea [15]. Despite the irregularly irregular vaginal bleeding reported with ENG implant use, a Brazilian study showed a 0.6 g/dL increase in Hb and 1.5 % in Hct among 37 female adolescents, aged 16–19 years, during implant use compared to those not using contraception. The study concluded this increase was probably due to amenorrhea and reduced bleeding volume or frequency of periods [19].

CONTRACEPTIVE EFFICACY AND EFFECTIVENESS

Half of the six million pregnancies in the United States each year are unintended or unplanned. Over a million of these six million pregnancies are terminated by elective abortion. The high rate of unintended pregnancies is not due to low efficacy of contraceptives, but to the challenges adolescents face in using methods correctly and consistently. The gap between perfect use and typical use increases with methods that are more user dependent, and adolescents represent a group with higher than usual failure rates for most user-dependent methods. The advantages of longer-acting contraceptives compared to combination methods are not only improved efficacy, safety, or acceptability, but also ease of use adaptable to the different cultural and lifestyle characteristics that make daily adherence difficult. Since higher risk behaviors are also more frequent among adolescents, it is appropriate to recommend a second method (e.g., dual method use) such as condoms to also prevent STI.

POPs: Effectiveness and Efficacy

Clinical studies with adults using POPs report 12-month pregnancy rates ranging from 1 to 13 % [4]. Typical-use failure rates of POPs are estimated at about 8–9 % per year with perfect-use failure rates at 0.3 % per year that is comparable to COCs [7]. A Cochrane Review of randomized controlled trials of POPs for contraception suggests superior efficacy of desogestrel compared to levonorgestrel pills, but the difference was small and only found in women who were not breast feeding. This review also suggested a failure rate for desogestrel pills that is comparable to COCs of 0.1 pregnancies per 100 woman-years [20]. The Cochrane Review could not draw any firm conclusions and suggested further research. POPs require strict adherence to taking each POP at the same time of the day, with only a 3-h window of variation. This adherence may be particularly challenging for adolescent and college-aged women; lack of consistent and correct use is a common cause of unintended pregnancy with POPs. There is no data to support decreased efficacy of POPs based on weight and dosage adjustment is not needed.

DMPA: Effectiveness and Efficacy
With perfect use, DMPA is highly effective with failure rates ranging from 0 to 0.3 % in the first year of use. This rate is the weighted average of failure rates in seven clinical trials i.e., 0.3 % when no more than 1 or 2 weeks late for a next injection. Even though initial estimates of the effectiveness (typical failure rate) of this method were similar to perfect-use efficacy, in 1995 the NSFG reported that with typical use, the method has a failure rate of 3 %. With DMPA, there is a 2-week grace period from the subsequent injection due date, with decreasing contraceptive effectiveness if subsequent reinjection is given after 15 weeks from the last injection date. Massaging the site of injection is discouraged since this leads to faster absorption and decreased duration of effectiveness. An adolescent's weight does not influence its efficacy and dosage adjustment is not needed based on weight [8]. Although the total dose of DMPA is lower with DMPA-SC than the IM preparation (104 mg versus 150 mg), the efficacy and effect on the return of fertility are no different from those associated with DMPA-IM [3].

Etonogestrel Implant: Effectiveness and Efficacy
Long-acting contraceptive methods, such as the implant, are considered one of the most effective and safest ways to avoid repeated pregnancies in adolescents. From its introduction in 1998, the ENG implant has been used in more than 30 countries by more than 3.3 million women. It is a highly effective contraceptive system, with an annual failure rate below 1 % for up to 3 years after insertion. Darney and colleagues analyzed clinical data from 11 international Good Clinical Practice-compliant studies conducted in the United States, Chile, Europe, and Asia. Efficacy was determined with 923 healthy, sexually active women, 18–40 years of age, who were within 80–130 % of ideal body weight. The analysis showed no pregnancies while women had their implant in place. Six pregnancies occurred during the first 14 days after implant removal and were included in the calculation of the cumulative Pearl Index for women ≤35 years old: 0.38 (number of pregnancies per 100 woman-years of use or annual pregnancy rate) which is similar to other long-acting contraceptive methods, including sterilization. These pregnancies might be explained by the fact that, although the implant inhibits ovulation, substantial ovarian activity is still present. Estradiol levels remain low during the first month after implant insertion and slowly increase during the subsequent

6 months. Since FSH levels remain similar to those seen in the normal follicular phase, a return of ovulation and potential conception can occur shortly after removal of the implant. Because the women ranged from 80 to 130 % of ideal body weight, these trials cannot predict efficacy in obese adolescent ENG implant users [21]. Funk et al. also found that no pregnancies resulted while the ENG implant was in place in an open-label, single-treatment study that assessed efficacy and safety in 330 18- to 40-year-old American women who used the implant for a total of 474 woman-years. Post-treatment information provided by the women showed that 46 were not using any contraceptive method following implant removal. Of these 46 women, 11 became pregnant between 1 and 18.5 weeks after removal of the implant but the conception date in all of these cases was after the date of implant removal based on ultrasound or a serum pregnancy test [15].

PROGESTIN-ONLY CONTACEPTIVES: ADVERSE EFFECTS AND DISCONTINUATION RATES

Overall, side effects contribute to contraceptive discontinuation. Unscheduled bleeding is the greatest challenge for POC users and the most common reason for discontinuation in up to 25 % of users [4]. Appropriate counseling on anticipating and managing irregular bleeding can have an important impact on adolescent and young adult women's adherence to these methods, especially since menstrual irregularities may stabilize over a longer duration of treatment in the case of POPs and DMPA.

Adverse Effects and Discontinuation of Progestin-Only Pills

- *Irregular vaginal bleeding*: Irregular bleeding can be a frequent side effect of POPs in up to 25 % of users [4] and it is the main reason for discontinuation of this method. On the other hand, consistent use may lead to amenorrhea, a desired outcome for many adolescents.
- *Ovarian cysts*: Unlike COCs that consistently inhibit ovulation and functional ovarian cyst formation, POPs are associated to increased incidence of functional ovarian cyst formation or persistent follicles.
- *Ectopic pregnancy*: A higher incidence of ectopic pregnancy has been observed in women using POPs compared to those using other contraceptive methods, although the incidence among women using POPs is similar to the incidence for women not using any contraception.

- Other less frequent side effects associated with the use of POPs include headache, nausea, dizziness, breast tenderness, and mood swings. Reduced libido, acne, and dysmenorrhea have also been described.

Adverse Effects and Discontinuation in the Use of DMPA

- *Irregular vaginal bleeding*: Spotting lasting >7 days and irregular bleeding are most common during the first months of use with an incidence of 70 % in the first year of use, and 10 % in subsequent years (after 5 years 80 % of users are amenorrheic). Although rarely heavy (hemoglobin values rise in DMPA users), bleeding is the most common reason for DMPA discontinuation. Management can include short courses of non-steroidal anti-inflammatory drugs for 5–7 days or, for women with no contraindications to estrogen use, low-dose combined oral contraceptives or estrogen supplementation for 10–20 days [5].
- *Weight gain*: Reported in up to 54 % of adolescent DMPA users, weight gain leads to discontinuation of DMPA in up to 40 % of adolescents [22]. Most studies do not differentiate between the effect of lifestyle and the effect of hormone itself. Reported data previously suggested that weight gain may be associated with specific patient characteristics such as African American race or increased weight and BMI at the initiation of DMPA therapy [23]. More recently, reports suggested that adolescents and young adult females who gain >5 % body weight within 6 months of DMPA use are at risk for future weight gain with continued DMPA [24]. Bonny et al. reported that regardless of race and baseline obesity, if >5 % weight gain did not occur by 6 months of DMPA use, then the risk for future weight gain is reduced. Taken as a whole, findings in adolescents so far indicate that DMPA use associated with an increase in body weight of >5 % in the first 6 months of use predicts risk for continued excessive weight gain, but overall, weight gain is not found among all adolescents on DMPA and most DMPA users do not experience extreme weight gain on this method [25–27].
- *Bone Mineral Density (BMD)*: Medroxyprogesterone doses in DMPA inhibit LH surge and ovulation, creating a hypoestrogenic state. The negative impact of this action on BMD has drawn particular attention for adolescents who may not have reached peak bone mass. However, there is evidence that this loss of BMD loss is completely or partially reversible [28]. There are no data showing that women who used DMPA as adolescents are at increased risk of fracture compared with nonusers.

The black box issued in 2004 by the FDA stated it is unknown if the use of Depo-Provera® contraceptive Injection during adolescence or early adulthood will reduce peak bone mass and increase the risk for osteoporotic fracture later in life, stressing this loss in BMD might not be completely reversible. In response to this warning, supported by a review of findings thus far, Cromer et al., in their Position Paper of the Society for Adolescent Medicine, recommended continuing to prescribe DMPA to adolescent girls needing contraception with adequate explanation of benefits and potential risks [29]. They also recommended 1,300 mg calcium carbonate intake plus 400 IU vitamin D and daily exercise to all adolescents receiving DMPA, with a consideration of estrogen supplementation in those girls with osteopenia (or those who have not had a Bone Density Study but are at high risk for osteopenia) who are otherwise doing well on DMPA and have no contraindication to estrogen. The American College of Obstetricians and Gynecologists Committee on Adolescent Health states that concerns about bone loss should not limit the use of DMPA in adolescents. They should follow age appropriate recommendations for calcium and vitamin D supplementation. Estrogen supplementation and discontinuation at 2 years are not required (ACOG Committee opinion No. 415 [30]). Similarly, the WHO guidelines state with regard to bone health, there should not be any restriction in the use of DMPA for women aged 18–45 years who are otherwise eligible to use this contraceptive. WHO also recommends balancing risks and benefits on an individual basis if considering long term use of this method.

- *Mood changes*: In a review of the literature, Cromer et al. concludes that earlier studies (conducted in the 1970s) had cited an association between DMPA use and depressive symptoms, but these studies lacked proper baseline assessment of mood disorder symptoms in the study population. Overall the conclusion of this author's review is that DMPA has no apparent deleterious effect on mood [31].
- *Galactorrhea*: Although reported in adolescents using DMPA, galactorrhea is self-limited and infrequent [32].
- *Metabolic changes*: The impact of DMPA on glucose tolerance and insulin resistance is not clinically relevant in healthy women, although monitoring has been suggested in those with glucose intolerance and diabetes [8]. DMPA can cause an increase in LDL-C and a decrease in HDL-C. However, its impact is negligible and it can lower total cholesteraol and tryglicerides [8].

- *STI*: Due to cervical cytological changes, an association with increased risk for acquiring STIs has been proposed, in particular with Chlamydia Trachomatis. Literature, however, implies the risk is associated with sexual behavior [4]. More recently another study showed no evidence that DMPA use was associated with increased STI risk [33]. There is no evidence that DMPA is associated with an increased risk for acquisition of HIV [31].

Less frequent DMPA-associated side effects include: headaches (probably due to fluid retention), mastalgia (in up to 15–20 % of users), decreased libido, and nervousness. However, these data are not specific to adolescents.

Adverse Effects and Discontinuation in the Use of ENG Implant

ENG implants are generally well tolerated. Studies show better adolescent continuation rates with the implant compared to adults. In a study conducted in Brazil, Guazzelli et al. reported a 0 % implant 12-month discontinuation rate in adolescents, lower than that of 26 % in adults [19].

Changes in menstrual bleeding patterns: The ENG implant has an unpredictable bleeding pattern. This side effect is the most common and it is the main reason for discontinuation. There are no data comparing adult and adolescent bleeding patterns on implants. In a review from 11 clinical trials, changes in vaginal bleeding patterns in women, ages 18–40 years, were mainly amenorrhea (22.2 %) and infrequent (33.6 %), frequent (6.7 %), and/or prolonged bleeding (17.7 %). The authors noted that even though bleeding-spotting days were fewer than or comparable to those observed during the natural cycle, they occurred at unpredictable intervals. The bleeding pattern experienced during the first 3 months after insertion tended to predict future patterns for the majority of women [34]. A US, multicenter trial of 330, women ages 18–40 reported a 13.0 % removal rate for changes in bleeding pattern. Participants had a higher amount of blood loss during the first 3 months of the study that subsequently decreased. Of note, highest rates of discontinuating the ENG implant were during the first 8 months of use [15]. Discontinuation rates due to bleeding irregularities vary greatly according to different geographic areas; approximately 14 % in the United States and Europe compared to 4 % in Southeast Asia, Chile, and Russia. Since bleeding characteristics were comparable in these areas, studies conclude that geographical differences in expectations and acceptance of changes in bleeding patterns seem to be better explained by cultural and social differences than due to actual blood loss [21]. Since irregular bleeding is the main reason for discontinuation, it is recommended that clinicians discuss with adolescents and young adult women that expected irregular vaginal bleeding and its management even before, and reinforced shortly after, insertion of the implant to improve continuation rates. Management can be similar to that used with DMPA and can include short courses of non-steroidal anti-inflammatory drugs for 5–7 days or, for women with no contraindications to estrogen use, low-dose combined oral contraceptives or estrogen supplementation for 10–20 days [5].

- *Weight changes*: Although not a common reason for discontinuation, weight gain has been commonly associated with ENG implant. Labeling data reports a mean weight gain of 2.8 lb after 1 year of implant use and 3.7 lb after 2 years, with no clear association of the weight gain and the implant use. Studies report weight gain among approximately 12 % of adult ENG implant users. However, only 3.3 % of users cited weight gain as a reason for discontinuation [15]. Guazzelli et al. noted no significant weight change in their adolescent post-partum population after 1 year of implanon use [35]. Data reported by Funk et al. and Croxatto et al. found a mean increase in BMI from baseline to last measurement of 0.7–0.8 kg/m^2 in their 18- to 40-years-old study population [15, 36].
- *Headaches*: Trials found that headache reports are lower with adult and adolescent ENG implant users (21 %) than previously reported with levonorgestrel implants, and more importantly, headache does not represent a frequent cause of discontinuation (4.7 %) [8] Guazzelli et al. reported headache among 29.5 % of their adolescent study population, but none of their 44 participants had headache as a cause for discontinuation of this method [35]. Funk et al. supported these findings in their study [15].
- *Mood changes*: Drug labeling data cites a history of depression as a reason to show caution in using the ENG implant. Given the high risk of this mood disorder in the adolescent population, it should be considered but is not a contraindication to use. An international study conducted in women, ages 18–40 years old, showed an incidence of 5.8 % of emotional labilty leading to discontinuation of the implant in 2.3 % [21].
- *Ovarian cysts*: During the first year of ENG implant use, about 5–7 % of women may develop ovarian cysts that generally do not require medical intervention. The ENG implant does not suppress FSH levels, and ovarian follicles continue to be stimulated. If follicular development occurs, atresia of the follicle is sometimes delayed, and the follicle may continue to grow

beyond the size it would attain in a normal cycle. When the LH peak is abolished, these follicles do not ovulate. Generally, these enlarged follicles disappear spontaneously over the course of weeks (described in an average of 10 weeks in adult women studies) and rarely surgery may be required.

- *Blood pressure*: Both literature and drug labeling data suggests safe use of the implant with close monitoring in well- controlled hypertension. Studies performed in adolescents showed blood pressure remained unchanged or within the normal range.

- *Lipid profile and insulin resistance*: ENG implant labeling states the implant may induce mild insulin resistance and small changes in glucose concentrations of unknown clinical significance. Literature supports there are no significant clinical effects of implants on carbohydrate metabolism or lipid profiles in implant users. In a study conducted in Brazil, 37 adolescents (mean age 17.2 years old) showed no significant changes in fasting glucose levels after 1 year of implant use. This lack of change was attributed to the low androgenic potential and the slow release of ENG. This same study found that the ENG implant improved the lipid profile in their users: reduction in total cholesterol (TC), Low Density Lipoprotein (LDL-C), VLDL-C (very low density lipoprotein), and TG (triglycerides). There were consequent increase in the HDL-C/TC and HDL-C/LDL-C ratios, with a reduction in risk for dyslipidemias. Similar findings were reported in a prospective, randomized, open pilot study that collected clinical and metabolic data in 18–35 years old post-partum exclusively breast-feeding mothers in Sao Paulo, Brazil [19]. This data is similar to that reported in adults [16].

- *Effect on liver function (increases in transaminases and bilirubin)*: Studies show mixed results, although overall changes in liver function tests are clinically insignificant [15,19]. Nevertheless, these changes should be taken into account in women with baseline hepatic conditions.

- *Complications of Insertion and Removal*: The single-rod implant is easily placed and removed and complications are rare. Prescribing information cites possible complications related to implant insertion and removal (pain, paresthesias, bleeding, hematoma, scarring, or infection in the insertion site) as well as local discomfort and pain experienced during and/or after insertion (reported by 2.9 % of women in clinical trials [Implanon® prescribing information]). If the implant is inserted too deeply (intramuscularly or in the fascia), the following may occur: neural or vascular injury, migration of the implant, and in a very few cases intravascular insertion and difficult removal requiring a surgical procedure for better location. Failure to insert the implant properly may go unnoticed unless it is palpated immediately after insertion. The Nexplanon® implant system contains barium to assist in locating the implant if removal is difficult or there is a question regarding location of the implant.

- *Acne*: Funk et al. [15] reported acne in 16.7 % of their 315 female participants, ages 18–40 years. Regardless whether participants reported having acne at baseline or not, post-treatment data showed unchanged or decreased incidence of acne. There is no data on the impact of the ENG implant on acne in younger adolescents.

Other adverse reactions reported as common (≥10 %): The most common adverse reactions reported in clinical trials were headache (24.9 %), vaginitis (14.5 %), weight increase (13.7 %), acne (13.5 %), breast pain (12.8 %), abdominal pain (10.9 %), and pharyngitis (10.5 %). Other potential risks reported include dysmenorrhea, the possibility of ectopic pregnancy, and interaction with antiepileptic drugs.

CONTRAINDICATIONS TO POCS

There are few serious risks associated with the use of POCs. The Centers for Disease Control in their 2010 Medical Eligibility Criteria list conditions for which use of POCs may represent unacceptable health risks (Category 3 or 4 recommendations-[Appendix A]). However, it is important to note that most of these recommendations are based on CHC, and the US MEC states it is not clear if they are the same for POCs (see Box 3.1). These conditions include:

Box 3.1 Contraindications to POCs

- Breast cancer
- Stroke
- Cardiovascular disease* (or multiple risk factors for it, such as older age, smoking, diabetes and hypertension)
- Hypertension: systolic ≥160 mmHg or diastolic ≥100 mmHg* or with associated vascular disease*
- Current and h/o ischemic heart disease
- Systemic lupus erythematosus with positive or unknown antiphospholipid antibodies
- Unexplained vaginal bleeding (before evaluation)*

*US MEC Category 3 for DMPA and category 2 for POPs and the implant.

In summary, POCs have been available for contraception for more than five decades in oral formulations, with more recently developed routes of administration that enhance efficacy by relying less on user adherence. POCs provide female adolescents with both contraceptive and non-contraceptive benefits, without the estrogenic effects that can cause unwanted side-effects seen with combination methods. The more potent progestins can be used at lower doses and can be delivered via oral, intramuscular, subcutaneuous, or subdermal long-acting delivery systems. The three POCs marketed in the United States that were discussed in this chapter offer adolescent and young adult women short- or long-acting, convenient, discreet, estrogen-free, and cost-effective contraceptive options. Female adolescents have unique contraceptive needs inherent to their age, psychosocial development, and socio-economic status resulting in their having difficulty effectively utilizing more user dependent contraceptive methods. In addition, POCs have a unique niche in serving the contraceptive needs of adolescent and young adult women, especially those who have medical contraindications to estrogens or medical conditions such as sickle cell disease or epilepsy that particularly benefit from DMPA. POCs are a particularly beneficial option for a subpopulation of adolescent and young adult women who need a safe, reversible, effective alternative to combination estrogen and progestin contraceptives.

REFERENCES

1. Centers for Disease Control and Prevention. U.S. medical eligibility criteria for contraceptive use, 2010. MMWR. 2010;59(RR-4): 1–86.
2. Grove D, Hooper DJ. Doctor contraceptive-prescribing behavior and women's attitudes towards contraception: two European. J Eval Clin Pract. 2011;17(3):493–502.
3. Ahrendt HJ, Adolf D, Buhling KJ. Advantages and challenges of estrogen-free hormonal contraception. Curr Med Res Opin. 2010;26(8):1947–55.
4. Hatcher RA, Trussell J, Nelson AL, Cates Jr W, Stewar FH, Kowal D. Contraceptive technology. 19 revisedth ed. New York: Contraceptive Technology Communications, Inc.; 2007.
5. Centers for Disease Control and Prevention. U.S. selected practice recommendations for contraceptive use, 2013. MMWR. 2013; 62(5):1–64.
6. Fritz M, Speroff L. Clinical gynecologic endocrinology and infertility. 8th ed. Philadelphia, PA: Lippincott Williams & Wilkins; 2011.
7. WHO. Medical eligibility criteria for contraceptive use. 4th ed. Geneva: WHO; 2009.

8. Neinstein LS, Gordon CM, Katzman DK, Rosen DS, Woods ER. Adolescent health care. A practical guide. 5th ed. Philadelphia, PA: Lippincott Williams & Wilkins; 2008.

9. Nelson AL, Katz T. Initiation and continuation rates seen in 2-year experience with same day injections of DMPA. Contraception. 2007;75(2):84–7. Epub 2006 31 Oct.

10. Rickert VI, Tiezzi L, Lipshutz J, León J, Vaughan RD, Westhoff C. Depo now: preventing unintended pregnancies among adolescents and young adults. J Adolesc Health. 2007;40(1):22–8.

11. Manchikanti Gomez A, Grimes DA, Lopez LM; Schultz KF. Steroid hormones for contraception in women with sickle cell disease. Cochrane Database Syst Rev. 2007;(2):CD006261.

12. Mattson RH, Cramer JA, Darney PD, Naftolin F. Use of oral contraceptives by women with epilepsy. JAMA. 1986;256:238–40.

13. Mattson RH, Rebar RW. Contraceptive methods for women with neurologic disorders. Am J Obstet Gynecol. 1993;168:2027–32.

14. Mosher WD, Jones J. Use of contraception in the United States: 1982–2008. Vital Health Stat. 2010;23(29):1–44.

15. Funk S, Miller MM, Mishell Jr DR, Archer DF, Poindexter A, Schmidt J. Safety and efficacy of Implanon, a single-rod implantable contraceptive containing etonogestrel. Contraception. 2005;71(5):319–26.

16. Brito MB, Ferriani RA, Quintana SM, Yazlle ME, de Sá Silva MF, Vieira CS. Safety of the etonogestrel releasing implant during the immediate postpartum period: a pilot study. Contraception. 2009;80:519–26.

17. Lewis L, Doherty D, Hickey M, Skinner AR. Implanon as a contraceptive choice for teenage mothers: a comparison of contraceptive choices, acceptability and repeat pregnancy. Contraception. 2010;81(5):421–6.

18. Yisa SB, Okenwa AA, Husemeyer RP. Treatment of pelvic endometriosis with etonogestrel subdermal implant (Implanon®). J Fam Plan Reprod Health Care. 2005;31:67–9.

19. Guazzelli CA, de Queiroz FT, Barbieri M, Torloni MR, de Araujo FF. Etonogestrel implant in postpartum adolescents: bleeding pattern, efficacy and discontinuation rate. Contraception. 2010; 82(3):256–9. Epub 2010 29 Mar.

20. Grimes DA, Lopez LM, O'Brien PA, Raymond EG. Progestin-only pills for contraception. Cochrane Database Syst Rev. 2010;(1):CD007541.

21. Darney P, Patel A, Rosen K, Shapiro L, Kaunitz A. Safety and efficacy of a single-rod etonogestrel implant (Implanon): results from 11 international clinical trials. Fertil Steril. 2009;91(5):1646–53. Epub 2008 18 Apr.

22. Harel Z, Biro FM, Kollar LM, Rauh JL. Adolescents' reasons for and experience after discontinuation of the long-acting contraceptives Depo-Provera and Norplant. J Adolesc Health. 1996;19(2):118–23.

23. Bonny AE, Britto MT, Huang B, et al. Weight gain, adiposity, and eating behaviors among adolescent females on depot medroxyprogesterone acetate (DMPA). J Pediatr Adolesc Gynecol. 2004; 17:109–15.

24. Le YC, Rahman M, Berenson AB. Early weight gain predicting later weight gain among depot medroxyprogesterone acetate users. Obstet Gynecol. 2009;114(2 Pt 1):279–84.

25. Bonny AE, Ziegler J, Harvey R, et al. Weight gain in obese and nonobese adolescent girls initiating depot medroxyprogesterone, oral contraceptive pills, or no hormonal contraceptive method. Arch Pediatr Adolesc Med. 2006;160:40–5.

26. Bonny AE, Secic M, Cromer B. Early weight gain related to later weight gain in adolescents on depot medroxyprogesterone acetate. Obstet Gynecol. 2011;117(4):793–7.

27. Risser WL, Gefter LR, Barratt MS, Risser JM. Weight change in adolescents who used hormonal contraception. J Adolesc Health. 1999;24(6):433–6.

28. Harel Z, Johnson CC, Gold MA, Cromer B, Peterson E, Burkman R, et al. Recovery of bone mineral density in adolescents following the use of depot medroxyprogesterone acetate contraceptive injections. Contraception. 2010;81(4):281–91. Epub 2009 14 Dec.

29. Cromer B. WHO-statement on hormonal contraception and bone health. Special program of research, development and research training in human reproduction (2005). J Adolesc Health. 2006;39(2):296–301.

30. American College of Obstetricians and Gynecologists. ACOG Committee Opinion No. 415: Depot medroxyprogesterone acetate and bone effects. Obstet Gynecol. 2008;112:727–30.

31. Cromer BA. Recent clinical issues related to the use of depot medroxyprogesterone acetate (Depo-Provera). Curr Opin Obstet Gynecol. 1999;11(5):467–71.

32. Cromwell P, Anyan W. Depot medroxyprogesterone acetate galactorrhea. J Adolesc Health. 1998;23(2):61. Reprod. 1999;14(4):976–81. doi:10.1093/humrep/14.4.976.

33. Romer A, Shew M, Gilliam M, Ofner S, Fortenberry JD. The effect of depo provera medroxy progesterone acetate on sexually transmitted infection acquisition. J Adolesc Health. 2012; Epub 5 June 2012.

34. Mansour D, Korver T, Marintcheva-Petrova M, Fraser IS. The effects of Implanon on menstrual bleeding patterns. Eur J Contracept Reprod Health Care. 2008;13(1):13–28.

35. Guazzelli C, Queiroz F, Barbieri M, Barreiros FA, Torloni MR, Araujo FF. Metabolic effects of contraceptive implants in adolescents. Contraception. 2011;84(4):409–12. Epub 2011 23 Mar.

36. Croxatto HB, Urbancsek J, Massai R, Bennink HC, Van Beek A, and the Implanon® Study Group*. A multicentre efficacy and safety study of the single contraceptive implant Implanon®. Hum Reprod. 1999;14(4):976–81. doi:10.1093/humrep/14.4.976.

Chapter 4
Combined Hormonal Contraception

Mimi Zieman

INTRODUCTION

While the adolescent female may resemble an adult physically, her lifestyle is quite different from an adult's, and consequently, helping her choose a contraceptive is a very different process than counseling adults. Important factors to consider for the adolescent include her level of independence, economic resources, plans for the future, cognitive and emotional development, understanding of her body and sexuality, influence of her family and partner, and consequences of an unintended pregnancy. The ability to access, or consent to an abortion, may be limited. Given both life stage, autonomy, finances, and consent issues, the consequences of an unintended pregnancy are much more serious and complex.

According to the National Survey of Family Growth, a government-sponsored national population survey, 96 % of teenagers (15–19years old) who are sexually active have used a contraceptive at some time. In the survey covering the time period 2006–2010, 96 % of females reported having ever used a condom. Other methods ever used by adolescents included withdrawal (57 %), oral contraceptives (56 %), depot medroxyprogesterone acetate (20 %), the patch (10 %), and the ring (5 %). Fifteen percent had ever used periodic abstinence or the "rhythm" method and 14 % reported using emergency contraception [1].

M. Zieman, M.D. (✉)
SageMed, 655 Idlewood Drive, Atlanta, GA 30327, USA
e-mail: mimizieman@gmail.com

A. Whitaker and M. Gilliam (eds.), *Contraception for Adolescent and Young Adult Women*, DOI 10.1007/978-1-4614-6579-9_4,
© Springer Science+Business Media New York 2014

This chapter discusses the use of combined oral contraceptives (COCs), the contraceptive vaginal ring (NuvaRing®), and the contraceptive patch (Ortho Evra®) in the adolescent population.

FORMULATIONS AND CYCLES OF COMBINED HORMONAL CONTRACEPTION

COCs vary in formulation; the dose of ethinyl estradiol (EE) ranges from 10 to 50 μg and uses a variety of progestins. More recently a COC containing estradiol valerate has been marketed. Some pills are monophasic having the same dose of hormones in each active pill and some are multiphasic varying the dose depending on the day of the cycle. Most pills are taken in a 28-day cycle in which up to 7 pills in the package contain no hormones ("placebo" pills). Withdrawal bleeding occurs while taking the placebo pills. Some COCs are available with longer, extended cycles. These pills are packaged with 84 active pills and 7 placebo pills (one formulation has 7 days of low-dose EE in the "placebo" pills) so that a scheduled withdrawal bleed occurs every 3 months. One COC is packaged for continuous use with 28 combined hormonal pills in the package. The disadvantage of using pill packages not labeled for extended use (i.e., containing only 21 active pills per package) is that insurance may not allow for early prescription refill or the coverage of the extra packs necessary to accomplish continuous use. When taken continuously, there is no scheduled withdrawal bleed. Many COC formulations can be used for extended cycling whereby the user skips the hormone-free pills. The advantages of continuous pill use include convenience of skipping a menstrual period and eliminating the symptoms that may occur during the hormone-free interval such as headaches, bloating, and dysmenorrhea [2, 3].

The NuvaRing® is a flexible plastic ring 5.4 cm in diameter and 4 mm in thickness. It has a steady-state release of 120 μg of etonogestrel and 15 μg of ethinyl estradiol daily. It is designed to be placed in the vagina and remain for 3 weeks followed by removal for 1 week to allow for a withdrawal bleed. It contains sufficient hormones to be left in place for 4 full weeks, then removed and replaced with a new device on the same day if the user wants to create an extended cycle (off-label use). Women who extend cycles of the ring experience fewer scheduled periods but more breakthrough bleeding [4]. Women who are extending their ring cycles and have prolonged unscheduled bleeding may benefit from removal of the ring for 4 days to allow for a withdrawal bleed [5].

The Ortho Evra® patch is a flexible, thin patch 20 cm². Each patch releases 150 μg norelgestromin and 20 μg ethinyl estradiol daily and is designed to be worn for 7 days. It can be worn on the upper arm, buttocks, lower abdomen, or torso (excluding the breasts). It is designed to be changed weekly for 3 weeks followed by a patch-free week during which withdrawal bleeding occurs. Extended use (84days) of the patch was studied in a trial in which 239 women were randomized to extended versus cyclic use of the patch. Median numbers of bleeding or spotting days were similar for both regimens, but extended use delayed the median time to first bleeding to 54 days versus 25 days. Satisfaction was high with both regimens [6]. There are no published data evaluating long-term risks of extended patch use.

MECHANISM OF ACTION

COCs, the patch, and the ring all work primarily by inhibiting ovulation. The hormonal progestin component suppresses the release of gonadotropin-releasing hormone (GnRH) from the hypothalamus and the luteinizing hormone (LH) surge from the pituitary. The estrogen potentiates the effects of the progestin by suppressing the release of follicle-stimulating hormone (FSH) from the pituitary contributing to inhibition of ovulation. In addition, the progestin has secondary affects including thickening the cervical mucus thereby inhibiting sperm penetration.

CHC also affects other parts of the reproductive tract. Progestins slow tubal motility which may disrupt ovum or embryo transport. CHC induces endometrial changes including atrophy, edema, and vascular changes which may affect implantation; however, since unintended pregnancies do occur—we also know that this is not the primary mechanism of action, and the endometrium can still support implantation.

CONTRACEPTIVE EFFICACY AND EFFECTIVENESS

The percent of women who experience an unintended pregnancy when using the pill, patch, or ring perfectly during the first year of use is 0.3 % or 3 per 1,000 women. However, the statistic for "typical use" should be added in counseling. The probability of an unintended pregnancy over the first year of typical use is 9 % [7]. For teenagers, pregnancy rates in the range of 30–38 % during first year of use have been reported [8, 9]. This large discrepancy between perfect and typical use is due to the difficulty users experience in adhering to perfect use of these methods. One study that used an electronic pill package to track use found that although women reported successful use in their diaries, adherence was poor and did not improve with time. During the third cycle of use, 54 % of users missed 3 or more active pills [10]. Furthermore, research on counseling interventions to improve successful use has not demonstrated improved effectiveness [11]. One useful intervention studied is providing multiple packs of pills at one visit, because obtaining monthly refills may be a barrier to successful use. In one study, dispensing a one-year supply of pills was associated with a 30 % reduction in the pregnancy rate compared with a one- or three-month supply [12].

Patch users weighing more than 90 kg or 198 lb in clinical trials had an increased risk of pregnancy. While the patch may still be chosen by obese women, they should be counseled about this possible risk, effective alternatives, and whether they will use a backup method such as condoms concurrently as well as their increased risk of VTE [13].

Given the high typical use failure rates of CHC in teenagers, long-acting reversible contraceptives (LARC) are better options for teenagers and use should be encouraged. The American Congress of Obstetricians and Gynecologists (ACOG) supports use of LARC as first-line methods of contraception to reduce unintended pregnancy rates [14] and supports use as safe and appropriate for adolescents [15].

SIDE EFFECTS

Adolescents also cite side effects as a reason for discontinuing CHC. In one study of adolescents who chose COC use postpartum or post-abortion, 46 % of users discontinued use by 6–18 months, mostly citing side effects [16]. Adolescents often worry about how their method affects weight [17] and acne. In one study, 37 % discontinued COCs due to perceived weight gain, yet this group gained no more weight than continuers who did not perceive weight change (14 %) [17]. A systematic review of whether combination methods cause weight gain found insufficient evidence but ruled out any large effect [18]. Although side effects are often blamed for discontinuation, several placebo-controlled randomized trials have found that the incidence of side effects commonly associated with COCs is found at the same rate in the placebo comparator group [19, 20]. In an RCT of 76 adolescents using COCs or placebo for dysmenorrhea, investigators found similar number and types of side effects in both groups [21].

The main side effect directly attributable to CHC is menstrual cycle changes. Teenagers should be counseled that they may experience unscheduled bleeding and that this side effect improves with time. Missing pills causes unscheduled bleeding, and smoking increases the risk. Lower-dose COCs such as 20 μg EE formulations are associated with more unscheduled bleeding than pills with >20 μg estrogen [22]. Using COCs will lessen menstrual bleeding significantly, and users can be instructed to skip placebo periods to achieve extended cycles and eliminate periods when desired.

Other side effects associated with hormones include breast tenderness and nausea, which are more common and severe with higher-dose formulations. More rare associations include melasma. Less specific side effects include headaches, mood changes, decreased libido, and weight changes. However, the incidence of these nonspecific side effects was no greater in treatment groups compared to placebo in controlled trials. It has been suggested that counseling patients to expect these side effects can make them more likely to occur [23]. See counseling section for expanded discussion of this issue.

Hormonal side effects are mostly the same for the pill, ring, and the patch. Patch users may experience local skin reactions at the patch site and ring users may experience increased vaginal discharge but no increased risk of vaginal infections.

CONTINUATION

One-year continuation rates for CHC initiators are cited as 67 % [7]. However, adolescent continuation rates are lower, with many studies finding more than 50 % of users discontinuing pills by 6 months [24, 25]. In one study, 42 % of COC users who discontinued their pills did not consult their clinician and 69 % of discontinuers not wishing to become pregnant switched to a less effective method such as condoms or no method at all [26].

One recent trial considered whether starting the pill on the day the adolescent was seen in the clinic (Quick Start), as opposed to conventional "Sunday start," would increase successful use in adolescents 12–17 years of age. Only 26 % of subjects were continuing use at 6 months regardless of Quick Start or conventional Sunday start despite being cared for in specialty clinics for adolescents. In addition, 8.3 % of subjects were pregnant by 6 months of study [27].

Some studies have enrolled postpartum adolescents to assess method use, continuation, and repeat pregnancy. While this particularly vulnerable population has demonstrated unintended pregnancy and therefore a problem with contraception in the past—they also may be more highly motivated to prevent another pregnancy. Polaneczky and colleagues enrolled adolescent mothers <17 years of age and compared postpartum use of

Norplant with COCs, with follow-up for a mean of 15 months. At follow-up, 95 % of Norplant users continued use compared with 33 % of pill users. In fact, 24 % of pill users never filled their prescription. Of those who initially planned to use COCs, 26 % used no method, 21 % switched to Norplant, 17 % condoms, and 2 % DMPA. During follow-up, 38 % (19/50) of those who planned to use COCs and 2 % (1/48) of those who chose Norplant became pregnant [8].

A more recent study followed postpartum teenagers, 11–19 years old, who chose COCs, the patch, or DMPA after delivery. At 1 year they found approximately 50 % continuing use of the pill or patch with a 30 % repeat pregnancy rate and 67 % still using DMPA with a 14 % pregnancy rate [9]. Despite a trend toward more successful use of the patch by teenagers in earlier research, this study found equally low continuation and high pregnancy rates with use of the pill or patch.

Some earlier studies found that teenagers are more successful using the once-a-week patch or the once-a-month ring than using the pill requiring daily adherence [28]. However, a recent study of pill, patch, ring, and DMPA use by adolescents and young women showed disheartening results. They enrolled 1,387 participants, 15–24 years old, and followed them prospectively for 1 year. Continuation rates were low for all methods: pills 32.7, ring 29.4, patch 10.9, and DMPA 12.1 per 100 women years. The pregnancy rates were also high: patch 30.1, ring 30.5, pill 16.5, and DMPA 16.1 per 100 women years [29].

In a comparative clinical trial of the pill and the ring in 273 college students, mean age 22 years old, despite high rates of adherence during the study period, only 26 % of ring users and 29 % of pill users were still using their method at 6 months following trial. Almost half of both groups were using condoms or no method citing inability to pay for the method as the most common reason for discontinuation [30].

These and other studies point to the challenge adolescents have with the adherence requirements of using CHCs and the importance of women choosing long-acting methods. This point is being corroborated in the Contraceptive Choice study. In that prospective cohort of 9,256 women from the St. Louis area, 86 % of users were still using a LARC method at 1 year compared with 56 % of users of short-term methods. In addition, short-term method users were 20 times more likely to get pregnant than users of LARC methods during the study. When the analysis was limited to subjects 14–19 years old, the 12-month continuation rate for LARC methods was 81 %, versus 44 % for short-term methods. At the end of 12 months, 75 % reported satisfaction with LARC methods versus 42 % users of non-LARC methods [31].

CONTRAINDICATIONS

Although there are few contraindications to CHC use, there are relatively more compared to progestin-only methods, IUDs, and barrier methods. Although many of the serious adverse events are less common in the adolescent and young adult population, a few deserve discussion here: venous thromboembolism, migraine headache, and smoking. See Appendix B for a full list of conditions for which CHC is contraindicated.

The overall risk of venous thromboembolism (VTE) is generally estimated as approximately twofold higher in users of CHC than in nonusers. The background incidence in women of reproductive age not using CHC is approximately 5–10 per 10,000 women years [32]. The increased risk is age related and, thus, lower in adolescents. One study reported a rate of 2.1 DVT per 10,000 women years of use in adolescents 14–19years old versus 9.2 in women 35–39years old [33]. There is continued controversy as to whether certain CHC products have additional increased risk of VTE. The patch, drospirenone-containing pills, and desogestrel-containing products have specific information in the prescribing information warning of a possible increase in risk of VTE. Despite the increased relative risk, the absolute risk of VTE remains very low and even lower for adolescent users.

Although the risk of VTE with any CHC use is lower than the risk during pregnancy, women and girls with a history of VTE should generally not use any type of CHC. The US MEC gives CHC a category 4 (unacceptable health risk) for women of any age with an acute deep vein thrombosis or pulmonary embolism (DVT/PE) or a history of DVT/PE with high risk of recurrence. For women with lower risk of recurrence, use of CHC gets a US MEC category 3 meaning risks outweigh benefits and should not use the method unless clinical judgment dictates otherwise. These category assignments are not modified if a woman is using anticoagulant therapy. For superficial thrombophlebitis, US MEC gives a category of 2 [34].

Migraine headache is a relatively common diagnosis in young women. It is estimated that 13 % of women 15–19years and 22 % of those 20–24years report having had migraines currently or in the past [35]. Although the evidence remains mixed regarding the use of CHC with migraine headaches, the US MEC assigns a category 4 to CHC use in the context of migraine headache with aura at any age. Because the diagnosis of aura can be difficult, consultation with a neurologist may be helpful. With no aura, for women under 35, initiation of CHC is given a category 2 (benefits outweigh risks), but if migraines develop while using CHC, the US MEC gives continuation of CHC use a category 3 (risks outweigh benefits).

All women and girls who smoke should be encouraged to quit. Although risks of cardiovascular events in adolescents are almost negligible, smoking increases risks and these risks are compounded by CHCs. However, the US MEC gives a category 2 for CHC use with any quantity of smoking for women under the age of 35.

Use of CHC in the context of adolescents with medical illness is discussed in detail in Chap. 9.

> *The risks of not using a contraceptive, with the possibility of unintended pregnancy, greatly outweigh the risks of CHC use.*

ADVANTAGES AND DISADVANTAGES OF CHC USE

Advantages
- Not associated with weight gain.
- Improves acne and hirsutism.
- Reduced premenstrual syndrome (PMS) symptoms, especially with extended cycling.
- Reduces menstrual bleeding (amount and number of days) and dysmenorrhea.
- Users can control menstrual cycle by eliminating hormone-free intervals (pills, ring).
- No effect on future fertility and rapid reversibility.
- Reduced risk of PID and ectopic pregnancy.
- Reduced risk of ovarian and endometrial cancer.
- Reduced serious risks as compared with pregnancy.
- Patch and ring offer convenience of non-daily method.

Disadvantages
- Unscheduled bleeding—especially in first few cycles or with inconsistent use
- Bloating or feeling of weight gain due to hormonal or fluid changes
- Some drug interactions
- Decreased libido or possible mood changes

- No protection against STIs (adolescents should still be actively encouraged to use condoms for prevention of STIs and to have EC available)
- Nonspecific side effects such as nausea, breast tenderness, headaches
- Rare serious risks such as venous thromboembolism or adenocarcinoma of the cervix. Other risks include unintended pregnancy, hypertension (discussed below) and melasma

Some suggest a different approach to counseling about nonspecific side effects: Grimes and Schultz propose more "optimistic counseling." Since data from randomized placebo-controlled trials found no difference in incidence of "background side effects" such as headache, nausea, breast pain, weight gain, depressive symptoms, and breast symptoms, they advise against bringing them up when prescribing CHC. They state that the mention of side effects can have a "nocebo" effect which makes a side effect more likely to occur by creating expectation. This expectation in turn leads to discontinuation [23].

STARTING AND CONTINUING CHC
CHC may be used in adolescents for contraception, medical indications, or both. Common non-contraceptive indications include menstrual and hormonal regulation for those with polycystic ovary syndrome and hypothalamic amenorrhea as well as menstrual-related symptomatology such as dysmenorrhea. An additional benefit for this population is improvement of acne, which occurs with all formulations although only some pills are labeled for this as an indication.

A user may start the method at any time she can be reasonably sure she is not pregnant. If started within the first 5 days after start of menses, no backup is needed. She may start on the day she is seen in the office (Quick Start) or on the Sunday after the first day of menses. If started more than 5 days from the first day of her LMP, she needs to use a barrier method or abstain from sex for the next 7 days [36] (see Appendix C). It is not necessary to do a speculum or bimanual exam prior to initiating CHC [36, 37]. ACOG currently recommends that a sexually active adolescent has her first Papanicolaou smear at the age of 21. Screening for STIs, if indicated, can be done by urine testing or vaginal swab, without requiring a speculum exam.

All CHC methods may be started within the first 7 days of an abortion or miscarriage (first or second trimester), including immediately post-abortion. In the postpartum period, an update to the US MEC recommends waiting 21 days to start CHC for

Provider Tips

Demonstrate, if possible, how to follow the package and affix a sticker to track days of the week.

Ask the teenager to think of a reminder system that will help her remember to take the pill or to place the patch or ring, e.g., when brushing teeth or an alarm on her cell phone.

Provide multiple pill, patch, or ring packages if possible and write prescription with refills for 1 year.

Advise to call or return with any problems or questions.

Reassure that unscheduled bleeding may occur, gets better with time, and for pill users is minimized by taking pill at same time every day.

If unscheduled bleeding is problematic, she should contact you and she can be evaluated for causes and possibly switched to different formulation.

Remind to note their CHC use when seeing other clinicians and to discontinue use 1 month prior to major surgery that would require prolonged immobilization.

nonbreastfeeding women with low risk for VTE and 30 days for low-risk breastfeeding women. For all women with risk factors for VTE, the recommendation is to delay start of CHC until 42 days after delivery [34].

Compliance with daily, weekly, and monthly regimens can be challenging. The CDC's US Selected Practice Recommendations for Contraceptive Use, released in June 2013, has easy-to-follow algorithms for delayed start and other lapses in use for COCs (Fig. 4.1), patch (Fig. 4.2), and ring (Fig. 4.3) [36].

Specific Patch Instructions
- The first day of the first patch becomes "patch change day," e.g., Sunday. On the following Sunday, remove first patch and apply second new patch. Discard patch by folding on itself and placing in garbage—do not flush down toilet. Repeat the following

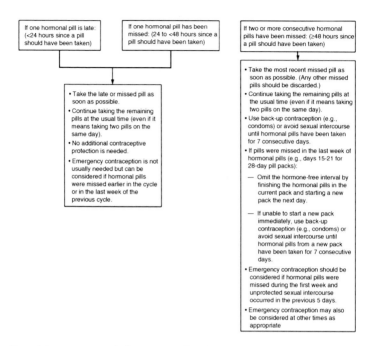

| If one hormonal pill is late: (<24 hours since a pill should have been taken) | If one hormonal pill has been missed: (24 to <48 hours since a pill should have been taken) | If two or more consecutive hormonal pills have been missed: (≥48 hours since a pill should have been taken) |

• Take the late or missed pill as soon as possible.
• Continue taking the remaining pills at the usual time (even if it means taking two pills on the same day).
• No additional contraceptive protection is needed.
• Emergency contraception is not usually needed but can be considered if hormonal pills were missed earlier in the cycle or in the last week of the previous cycle.

• Take the most recent missed pill as soon as possible. (Any other missed pills should be discarded.)
• Continue taking the remaining pills at the usual time (even if it means taking two pills on the same day).
• Use back-up contraception (e.g., condoms) or avoid sexual intercourse until hormonal pills have been taken for 7 consecutive days.
• If pills were missed in the last week of hormonal pills (e.g., days 15-21 for 28-day pill packs):
— Omit the hormone-free interval by finishing the hormonal pills in the current pack and starting a new pack the next day.
— If unable to start a new pack immediately, use back-up contraception (e.g., condoms) or avoid sexual intercourse until hormonal pills from a new pack have been taken for 7 consecutive days.
• Emergency contraception should be considered if hormonal pills were missed during the first week and unprotected sexual intercourse occurred in the previous 5 days.
• Emergency contraception may also be considered at other times as appropriate

Fig. 4.1 Recommended actions after late or missed combined oral contraceptives. Reprinted from [36].

week until patches have been worn for 3 weeks in a row. Remove third patch and do not wear a patch for a week. When this week is finished, start a new cycle.

• Patches may be placed on the upper arm, buttocks, abdomen, or torso (except on breasts). Apply to clean dry skin. Do not apply over any creams or it may not stick. Press firmly on patch for 10 s ensuring that the edges are well attached. Do not use any bandages to try to make patches stick better.
• Check the patch daily to ensure it continues to stick well. It can be worn while bathing, exercising and swimming.
• Detachment occurs with about 5 % patches. If a patch partially detaches for <24 h, the user should try to smooth it down. If it will not stick well, she should remove patch and replace with a new patch keeping her usual patch change day. If it has been >48 h or an unknown length of time, the patch

Delayed application or detachment* for <48 hours since a patch should have been applied or reattached	Delayed application or detachment* for ≥48 hours since a patch should have been applied or reattached

| • Apply a new patch as soon as possible. (If detachment occured <24 hours since the patch was applied, try to reapply the patch or replace with a new patch.)
• Keep the same patch change day.
• No additional contraceptive protection is needed.
• Emergency contraception is not usually needed but can be considered if delayed application or detachment occurred earlier in the cycle or in the last week of the previous cycle. | • Apply a new patch as soon as possible.
• Keep the same patch change day.
• Use back-up contraception (e.g., condoms) or avoid sexual intercourse until a patch has been worn for 7 consecutive days.
• If the delayed application or detachment occurred in the third patch week:
— Omit the hormone-free week by finishing the third week of patch use (keeping the same patch change day) and starting a new patch immediately.
— If unable to start a new patch immediately, use back-up contraception (e.g., condoms) or avoid sexual intercourse until a new patch has been worn for 7 consecutive days.
• Emergency contraception should be considered if the delayed application or detachment occurred within the first week of patch use and unprotected sexual intercourse occurred in the previous 5 days.
• Emergency contraception may also be considered at other times as appropriate. |

* If detachment takes place but the woman is unsure when the detachment occurred, consider the patch to have been detached for ≥ 48 hours since a patch should have been applied or reattached.

FIG. 4.2 Recommended actions after delayed application or detachment with combined hormonal patch. Reprinted from [36].

should be replaced and the user should use backup or abstain from sex for 7 days. Consider EC (Fig. 4.2).

• Skin reactions: patch locations should be rotated. Patches should not be placed over irritated skin.

Specific Ring Instructions

• Women should record what day they insert the ring so as to remember when to remove (3 weeks later) and when to insert a new ring (4 weeks later). The ring is inserted in the vagina and does not need a specific insertion technique or placement. Hormone levels provide protection for 35 days.

• Can be used with tampons (just be careful that ring doesn't fall out when removing tampon!)

• Users may experience vaginal symptoms such as discharge, feeling ring by partner during intercourse, or discomfort.

• Ring expulsion occurs in 6–9 % of users [38, 39]. Expulsion may occur during intercourse, a bowel movement, tampon removal, or other time. Rinse with lukewarm water and reinsert.

Delayed insertion of a new ring or delayed reinsertion* of a current ring for <48 hours since a ring should have been inserted	Delayed insertion of a new ring or delayed reinsertion* for ≥48 hours since a ring should have been inserted
• Insert ring as soon as possible. • Keep the ring in until the scheduled ring removal day. • No additional contraceptive protection is needed. • Emergency contraception is not usually needed but can be considered if delayed insertion or reinsertion occurred earlier in the cycle or in the last week of the previous cycle.	• Insert ring as soon as possible. • Keep the ring in until the scheduled ring removal day. • Use back-up contraception (e.g., condoms) or avoid sexual intercourse until a ring has been worn for 7 consecutive days. • If the ring removal occurred in the third week of ring use: — Omit the hormone-free week by finishing the third week of ring use and starting a new ring immediately. — If unable to start a new ring immediately, use back-up contraception (e.g., condoms) or avoid sexual intercourse until a new ring has been worn for 7 consecutive days. • Emergency contraception should be considered if the delayed insertion or reinsertion occurred within the first week of ring use and unprotected sexual intercourse occurred in the previous 5 days. • Emergency contraception may also be considered at other times as appropriate.

* If removal takes place but the woman is unsure of how long the ring has been removed, consider the ring to have been removed for ≥ 48 hours since a ring should have been inserted or reinserted.

FIG. 4.3 Recommended actions after delayed insertion or reinsertion with combined vaginal ring. Reprinted from [36].

US MEC DRUG INTERACTION RATINGS FOR CHC

CHC induces cytochrome P-450 enzyme activation and will cause more rapid clearance of drugs metabolized by this pathway. Therefore there is a short list of medications for which concurrent use with CHC is contraindicated (see Appendix B). The following medications are given a US MEC category 3 (risks outweigh benefits):

• Certain anticonvulsants: phenytoin, carbamazepine, barbiturates, primidone, topiramate, oxcarbazepine.
• Lamotrigine.
• Rifampin or rifabutin.
• Ritonavir-boosted protease inhibitors. For latest information on antiretrovirals, see http://aidsinfo.nih.gov/guidelines/html/1/adult-and-adolescent-treatment-guidelines/32/drug-interactions.

Of note, the commonly held belief that broad-spectrum antibiotics should not be used with CHC is not supported by the US MEC, which gives their use together a category 1 (no restrictions).

FOLLOW-UP

A follow-up appointment, usually for 3 months after initiation of CHC, is not necessary but is often recommended, especially for adolescents to assess their satisfaction and continuation of the method. However, there is no evidence to support this practice, and the decision to schedule a follow-up visit can be made on an individual basis [36]. Even if a follow-up is scheduled, a full year's contraception supply should be written at the initiation visit since she may not return for the follow-up visit. Blood pressure should be checked at the annual visit, since it can occasionally rise on CHC [36]. A large study found an incidence attributable to COCs of 41 cases per 10,000 women per year in 25–42-year-old women using a range of formulations [40].

Follow-up visits may address complaints women have and an opportunity to assess successful use. If troubled by adherence issues or other complaints, assess whether the adolescent would like to try a longer-acting method, which requires less attention than CHC. Providers should reinforce the need for protection from STIs and when to use EC.

ISSUES FOR ADOLESCENTS AND YOUNG WOMEN

1. Normal growth and development:
   There is concern that taking a CHC could disrupt normal development. However, if started after menarche in a cycling adolescent, use of CHC does not preclude normal function of the hypothalamic pituitary axis or precipitate early closure of the epiphyseal plates so does not stunt growth.
2. Bone effects:
   There are currently no restrictions on use of CHC in adolescents due to concerns about bone or development of bone density according to the CDC, WHO, or prescribing information.
3. Method choice:
   The goal of contraceptive selection is to find a method that suits the individual and that can be used successfully. Adolescents are more likely to discontinue CHC and to have challenges with regard to cost, transportation, and obtaining refills. CHC may be a particularly good choice for those with acne, PMS, and dysmenorrhea where the methods have particular benefits. Adolescents and providers must also consider that the "cost" of an unintended pregnancy is higher in this population. Young women should be counseled thoroughly, weighing these issues, and they should be apprised of the data that supports LARC as methods that teenagers are more successful with.

4. Choosing between pill, patch, and ring:

   In a systematic review of randomized controlled trials of women across all ages, the authors concluded that effectiveness was similar across all methods. The patch users had better adherence but more side effects than COC users which caused higher discontinuation. Ring users had fewer side effects such as breast discomfort and nausea than COC users, but more vaginal discharge [41].

5. Choosing a pill for acne:

   Is there a best pill for acne? According to the Cochrane systematic review of this topic, few significant differences were found in the COCs that were studied in placebo-controlled trials. One can generalize that due to the effects of CHC on reducing free testosterone and increasing sex hormone-binding globulin, all formulations are probably effective. COCs also prevent the conversion of free testosterone to dihydrotestosterone by blocking androgen receptors and inhibiting 5-alpha-reductase activity [42].

SUMMARY

Combination hormonal contraceptives are popular with adolescents because they are safe, effective, and easy to initiate and to discontinue. They have many non-contraceptive benefits uniquely desired by this population such as cycle control and reduction in acne. The suboptimal typical use effectiveness and high discontinuation rates are major drawbacks. Effective, tailored counseling needs to be done to find the method that enables success. Open nonjudgmental communication will encourage young women to return and discuss challenges.

REFERENCES

1. Martinez G, Copen CE, Abma JC. Teenagers in the United States: sexual activity, contraceptive use, and childbearing, 2006–2010 National Survey of Family Growth. Vital Health Stat 23. 2011;31:1–35.
2. Machado RB, de Melo NR, Maia H. Bleeding patterns and menstrual-related symptoms with the continuous use of a contraceptive combination of ethinylestradiol and drospirenone: a randomized study. Contraception. 2010;81:215–22.
3. Sulak PJ, Kuehl TJ, Ortiz M, Shull BL. Acceptance of altering the standard 21-day/7-day oral contraceptive regimen to delay menses and reduce hormone withdrawal symptoms. Am J Obstet Gynecol. 2002;186:1142–9.
4. Miller L, Verhoeven CH, Hout J. Extended regimens of the contraceptive vaginal ring: a randomized trial. Obstet Gynecol. 2005; 106:473–82.

5. Sulak PJ, Smith V, Coffee A, Witt I, Kuehl AL, Kuehl TJ. Frequency and management of breakthrough bleeding with continuous use of the transvaginal contraceptive ring: a randomized controlled trial. Obstet Gynecol. 2008;112:563–71.
6. Stewart FH, Kaunitz AM, LaGuardia KD, Karvois DL, Fisher AC, Friedman AJ. Extended use of transdermal norelgestromin/ethinyl estradiol: a randomized trial. Obstet Gynecol. 2005;105:1389–96.
7. Trussell J. Contraceptive failure in the United States. Contraception. 2011;83:397–404.
8. Polaneczky M, Slap G, Forke C, Rappaport A, Sondheimer S. The use of levonorgestrel implants for contraception in adolescent mothers. N Engl J Med. 1994;331:1201–6.
9. Thurman AR, Hammond N, Brown HE, Roddy ME. Preventing repeat teen pregnancy: postpartum depot medroxyprogesterone acetate, oral contraceptive pills, or the patch? J Pediatr Adolesc Gynecol. 2007;20:61–5.
10. Potter L, Oakley D, de Leon-Wong E, Canamar E. Measuring compliance among oral contraceptive users. Fam Plann Perspectives. 1996;28:154–8.
11. Halpern V, Lopez LM, Grimes DA, Gallo MF. Strategies to improve adherence and acceptability of hormonal methods of contraception. Cochrane Database Syst Rev. 2011;(4):CD004317.
12. Foster DG, Hulett D, Bradsberry M, Darney P, Policar M. Number of oral contraceptive pill packages dispensed and subsequent unintended pregnancies. Obstet Gynecol. 2011;117:566–72.
13. Zieman M, Guillebaud J, Weisberg E, Shangold GA, Fisher AC, Creasy GW. Contraceptive efficacy and cycle control with Ortho Evra: the analysis of pooled data. Fertil Steril. 2002;77:S13–8.
14. ACOG Committee Opinion Number 450. Increasing use of contraceptive implants and intrauterine devices to reduce unintended pregnancy. Obstet Gynecol. 2009;114:1434–8.
15. ACOG Committee Opinion Number 539. Adolescents and long-acting reversible contraception: implants and intrauterine devices. Obstet Gynecol. 2012;120:983–8.
16. Blumenthal PD, Wilson LE, Remsburg RE, Cullins VE, Huggins GR. Contraceptive outcomes among postpartum and post-abortal adolescents. Contraception. 1994;50:451–60.
17. Emans SJ, Grace E, Woods ER, Smith DE, Klein K, Merola J. Adolescents' compliance with the use of oral contraceptives. JAMA. 1987;257:3377–81.
18. Gallo MF, Lopez LM, Grimes DA, Schulz KF, Helmerhorst FM. Combination contraceptives: effect on weight. Cochrane Database Syst Rev. 2008;(4):CD003987.
19. Coney P, Washenik K, Langley RGB, DiGiovanna JJ, Harrison DD. Weight change and adverse event incidence with a low-dose oral contraceptive: two randomized, placebo-controlled trials. Contraception. 2001;63:297–302.

20. Redmond G, Godwin AJ, Olson W, Lippman JS. Use of placebo controls in an oral contraceptive trial: methodological issues and adverse event incidence. Contraception. 1999;60:81–5.
21. O'Connel K, Davis AR, Kerns J. Oral contraceptives: side effects and depression in adolescent girls. Contraception. 2007;75: 299–304.
22. Gallo MF, Nanda K, Grimes DA, Lopez LM, Schultz KF. 20microgram versus > 20mcg estrogen combined oral contraceptives for contraception. Cochrane Database Syst Rev. 2011;(1):CD003989
23. Grimes DA, Schultz KF. Nonspecific side effects of oral contraceptives: nocebo or noise? Contraception. 2011;83:5–9.
24. Berenson AB, Wiemann CM. Contraceptive use among adolescent mothers at 6 months postpartum. Obstet Gynecol. 1997;89:999–1005.
25. Oakley D, Sereika S, Bogue EL. Oral contraceptive pill use after an initial visit to a family planning clinic. Fam Plann Perspect. 1991;23:150–4.
26. Rosenberg MJ, Waugh MS. Oral contraceptive discontinuation: A prospective evaluation of frequency and reasons Am J Obstet Gynecol. 1998;179:577–82.
27. Edwards S, Zieman M, Jones K, Diaz A, Robilotto C, Westhoff C. Initiation of oral contraceptives—start now! J Adolesc Health. 2008;43:432–6.
28. Archer DF, Cullins V, Creasy GW, Fisher AC. The impact of improved compliance with a weekly contraceptive transdermal system (Ortho Evra) on contraceptive efficacy. Contraception. 2004;69:189–95.
29. Raine TR, Foster-Rosales A, Upadhyay UD, Boyer CB, Brown BA, Sokoloff A, Harper CH. One-year contraceptive continuation and pregnancy in adolescent girls and women initiating Hormonal Contraceptives. Obstet Gynecol. 2011;117:363–71.
30. Gilliam ML, Neustadt A, Kozloski M, Mistretta S, Tilmon S, Godfrey E. Adherence and acceptability of the contraceptive ring compared with the pill among students, a randomized controlled trial. Obstet Gynecol. 2010;115:503–10.
31. Rosenstock JR, Peipert JF, Madden T, Zhao Q, Secura GM. Continuation of reversible contraception in teenagers and young women. Obstet Gynecol. 2012;120(6):1298–305.
32. Heinemann LAJ, Dinger JC. Range of published estimates of venous thromboembolism incidence in young women. Contraception. 2007;75:328–36.
33. Obrien SH. Trends in prescribing patterns of hormonal contraceptives for adolescents. Contraception. 2008;77:264–9.
34. Centers for Disease Control and Prevention. Update to CDC's U.S. Medical Eligibility Criteria for Contraceptive Use, 2010: revised recommendations for the use of contraceptive methods during the postpartum period. MMWR Morb Mortal Wkly Rep. 2011;60(26):878–83.

35. Stewart WF, Wood C, Reed ML, Roy J, Lipton RB, AMPP Advisory Group. Cumulative lifetime migraine incidence in women and men. Cephalalgia. 2008;28(11):1170–8.
36. Centers for Disease Control and Prevention (CDC). U.S. Selected Practice Recommendations for Contraceptive Use, 2013. MMWR Recomm Rep. 2013;62(5):1–64.
37. Stewart FH, Harper CC, Ellertson CE, Grimes DA, Sawaya GF, Trussell J. Clinical breast and pelvic examination requirements for hormonal contraception: current practice vs. evidence. JAMA. 2001;285(17):2232–9.
38. Roumen FJ, op ten Berg MM, Hoomans EH. The combined contraceptive vaginal ring(NuvaRing): first experience in daily clinical practice in the Netherlands. European Journal of Contraception & Reproductive Health Care. 2006;11(1):14–22.
39. Veres L, Miller B, Burington A. Comparison between the vaginal ring and oral contraceptives. Obstet Gynecol. 2004;104:555–63.
40. Chasan-Taber L, Willett WC, Manson JE, Spiegelman D, Hunter DJ, Curhan G, Colditz GA, Stampfer MJ. Prospective study of oral contraceptives and hypertension among women in the United States. Circulation. 1996;94:483–9.
41. Lopez LM, Grimes DA, Gallo MF, Schulz KF. Skin patch and vaginal ring versus combined oral contraceptives for contraception. Cochrane Database Syst Rev. 2008;(1):CD003552.
42. Arowojolu AO, Gallo MF, Lopez LM, Grimes DA, Garner SE. Combined oral contraceptive pills for treatment of acne. Cochrane Database Syst Rev. 2009;(3):CD004425.

Chapter 5
Barrier Methods

Elisabeth Woodhams and Melissa Gilliam

INTRODUCTION

Condoms are the only contraceptive method that also protect against sexually transmitted infections (STIs). Contraceptive efficacy can approach a failure rate of 2 % per year if used perfectly; typical-use failure rate is about 17 % per year [1].

Historically, condoms have been strongly emphasized for adolescents and are the most commonly used contraceptive in this population. Condom use presents some unique challenges for teenaged women in that they are effective contraceptives [2] when used correctly but require participation from both partners. In spite of effective interventions that have increased condom use, perfect use remains elusive in this population and condom failure contributes to high rates of STIs and unintended pregnancy among teenaged women in this country.

In this chapter we discuss basic epidemiology of condom use among teenaged women and examine the contraceptive efficacy of condoms in this population. We explore the role of barrier methods in dual-method protection, discuss unique challenges and considerations young women face when engaging in condom use, and consider provider issues when discussing condom use. We will briefly touch on other barrier methods, specifically the female condom, as a possible alternative to male condoms for teenaged women.

E. Woodhams, M.D. (✉) • M. Gilliam, M.D., M.P.H.
Department of Obstetrics and Gynecology, Section of Family Planning and Contraceptive Research, The University of Chicago,
5841 S. Maryland Ave., MC 2050, Chicago, IL 60637, USA
e-mail: ewoodhams@uchicago.edu; mgilliam@babies.bsd.uchicago.edu

A. Whitaker and M. Gilliam (eds.), *Contraception for Adolescent and Young Adult Women*, DOI 10.1007/978-1-4614-6579-9_5,
© Springer Science + Business Media New York 2014

There are no medical contraindications to barrier birth control methods. However, these methods are associated with high typical-use failure rates. The 2010 Center for Disease Control (CDC) US Medical Eligibility Criteria (US MEC) for Contraceptive Use states that women with medical conditions associated with a high risk of adverse consequences from unintended pregnancy should be advised that sole use of barrier or behavioral methods may not be an appropriate choice due to high typical-use failure rates [3]. This is discussed in more detail in Chap. 9.

MALE AND FEMALE CONDOMS
Background/Epidemiology
Male Condoms

Male condoms are the most commonly used contraceptive among adolescents [2, 4]. In the most recent National Survey of Family Growth, 96 % of all females aged 15–19 had ever used a condom, far exceeding those who had ever used the oral contraceptive pill (56 %) [5]. There has been an overall rise in rates of condom use; in 1988 only 50 % of teenaged women reported having used a condom at first sex compared to 68 % in 2005 [5]. Contraceptive use at most recent intercourse has been used as a marker for regular contraceptive use, and 52 % of teenaged women say they used a condom at last intercourse; 49 % say they use a condom every time they have sex [5].

Patterns of use may vary by ethnicity and race. Hispanic adolescent women are less likely to have used a condom at last intercourse than non-Hispanic white or non-Hispanic black women in the same age group (47 % compared to 52 % and 58 %, respectively). Use also differs by age range, as older adolescents are more likely to have used a condom at last sex than their younger counterparts [5].

More recently, condoms have been supported for STI prevention rather than contraception in favor of other highly effective contraceptive methods [6]. In spite of this recommendation, 78 % of teenaged women say they use condoms primarily for contraception [7]. Teenagers may favor condoms as they are easier to obtain than other methods of contraception [4, 6] or may have concerns about confidentiality with healthcare providers [8].

Female Condoms

Female condoms are the only female-initiated barrier method of contraception, yet uptake in the United States has been slow [9]. There are no statistics on female condom use by adolescent women; the method is usually lumped within "other barrier methods" during large surveys [5] or ignored completely [10]. Acceptability is a significant barrier to female condom use [9]— most adult women prefer the male condom to female condom [5, 11]. There are few data on acceptability among teenagers [12]; a small survey study found acceptability was influenced by user discomfort placing the condom, as well as an overall preference for male condoms, even after an educational intervention [13]. Lack of access was also perceived as a barrier and the majority of participants stated that they would try them if they were available in spite of their discomfort with placing them [13].

Mechanism of Action
Male Condoms
There are a variety of male condoms; the most popular are made of latex. People with latex allergies can use polyurethane and silicone condoms. These condoms are very thin (0.8 mm thick at their greatest thickness) and impenetrable to sperm, as well as to the organisms that cause STIs and HIV [14, 15]. There is also some evidence that condoms prevent against HPV [15]. Natural skin condoms ("lambskin") are available, but do not prevent HIV and STIs and have higher rates of breakage [1].

Female Condoms
The female condom is made of polyurethane, latex or, most recently, nitrile.

Like the male condom, the female condom creates a physical barrier to prevent spillage of sperm and semen in to the vaginal canal [16]. The female condom has an outer ring, an inner ring, and the condom between the rings. Newer versions of the condom also have a vaginal sponge in the inner ring to assist in holding the condom in place. It is recommended that ample lubrication be applied to the inside of the condom prior to insertion to help decrease noise of the condom and also prevent slippage. There is one type of female condom FDA approved for use in this country (FC2 Female Condom®, previously Reality Female Condom®).

Contraceptive Efficacy
Male Condoms
When used correctly, male condoms are extremely effective at preventing pregnancy. Perfect use is associated with a failure rate of only 2 % in the first year. In contrast, typical-use failure approaches 17 % in the first year [1]. Age also factors into effective condom use, as older couples are generally more experienced,

more motivated to prevent pregnancy, and more likely to use condoms correctly and consistently [17].

Condom failures are largely attributed to misuse or problems with the condom itself. Condoms break from 1 to 8 times per 100 episodes of vaginal intercourse. In addition to breaking, the condom slips in 1–5 % of episodes. These numbers decrease with experience [18]. Lubricants can increase the risk of slippage or breakage; teens should be advised that all lubricants need to be water based as oil-based lubricants will weaken latex [1]. Spermicides decrease the risk of pregnancy if the condom slips or breaks, but all teens should be counseled to use emergency contraception as quickly as possible.

Many teenagers use condoms incorrectly. In a survey of teen university students, 38 % of respondents applied the condom after sex had begun, and 13 % removed it before sex was concluded [19]. Several others used a sharp instrument to open the package, which can compromise the integrity of the condom [17]. Teenagers should also be counseled about other factors that affect the condom, including the latex breakdown in condoms that are old or expired (consider the condom that has been safely kept in the wallet for a year). While preparedness is to be applauded, latex that has been kept in a warm environment begins to breakdown after more than a month, which increases the risk of condom breakage or slippage. If condoms are kept away from heat or humidity, they can be effective for 5 years [17].

Finally, breakage rates and failure rates appear to be higher with polyurethane condoms compared to latex condoms. Polyurethane condoms have breakage rates reported as high as 8 % [20], and in the Cochrane Review, the odds ratio of breakage for non-latex condoms ranges from 2.5 to 5 times that of the latex condoms [21].

Female Condoms
Studies of the female condom demonstrate that efficacy rates are slightly lower than for the male condom [6, 16, 22]. First-year failure rates range from 1 to 5 % for perfect use [22, 23] and 9 to 21 % for normal use [23, 24]. Like male condoms, the failure rates have been attributed to misuse, inconsistent use, and failure of the device [22].

Side Effects
Male and Female Condoms
A notable side effect of condoms relates to spermicides, which may be applied to certain types of male condoms. Spermicides are associated with increased colonization of the urinary tract with *E. coli* or *Staphylococcus saprophyticus* because of the change in the vaginal flora associated with their use [25–27]. Adolescents may also complain of vaginal irritation or itching related to condom use, which may be related to the presence of spermicides.

Continuation
Regular condom use declines rapidly as adolescent relationships become more serious or long standing; condom use is less consistent within 3 weeks of first sex within a relationship. In one study, up to 68 % of young women reported inconsistent condom use with their regular partner [27]. This change in condom use is thought to be related to a decrease concern for STIs as the relationship is perceived as more committed [5].

Contraindications
Latex allergy has a prevalence of 3–8.7 % in the general population [28]. It presents as a dermatitis-like rash or irritation most commonly; rarely latex allergy presents as anaphylaxis [28]. For adolescents who have latex allergy, condoms made of alternate materials are available (including polyurethane and silicone, as described above). Non-latex condoms are available; however, given that they are less efficacious, contraceptive providers should be certain that a patient has a latex allergy or sensitivity prior to recommending non-latex condoms [29].

Issues for Adolescents and Young Women
Predictors of condom use can inform providers about who might be at greater risk for misuse or nonuse. Younger age at first sex, older partner age, history of sexual abuse, obesity, and substance use are all predictors for condom nonuse among teens [22–26]. Young women also have a particularly challenging role in the negotiation of male condom use, as use requires complete cooperation from their partners. This challenge is also true for female condoms; although they are considered a female-initiated barrier method, they do require partner cooperation.

Counseling Considerations
An adolescent healthcare visit is a unique opportunity for reproductive health information and intervention, yet fewer than 30 % of healthcare providers provide condoms in their clinics, and less than 20 % provide education about their use [30]. Thirty percent of young women state that they do not get education about pregnancy prevention in schools [31], and in 2006 only 5 % of high schools made condoms available to students [32]. Therefore, it is prudent not to make assumptions about a patient's knowledge and include the basics, including explicit descriptions and examples of how to use both male and female condoms [31].

All male condoms are applied the same way, and healthcare providers should model application to help teenagers use them correctly. Providers should emphasize that to be effective a condom needs to be placed on the penis prior to any sexual contact with a partner and needs to remain on the penis throughout sexual intercourse. Air should be squeezed out of the top of the condom to create a reservoir, and the condom should then be rolled to the base of the shaft of the penis. The reservoir that was created should extend about a half inch from the end of the penis [1].

When removing the condom, the penis should first be removed completely from the vagina while still erect, and the condom held at the base to prevent spillage. The condom is then rolled down the penis [1].

Application of a female condom can be a more challenging task, but good education and practice decreases that barrier [9]. The woman gets in a comfortable position on her back or sitting down. The inner ring is squeezed and inserted into the vagina. She then places a finger through the condom and pushes the ring up to the top of the vagina. The outer ring should be flush with the outside of the vagina. The couple should be sure that the penis enters the condom and doesn't slip between the condom and the vagina.

To remove the condom, the woman should squeeze the outer ring shut to prevent spillage and gently pull the condom out (Fig. 5.1).

The timing of counseling about contraceptive use, especially condoms, is extremely important. Discussing condom use as part of a routine healthcare visit will increase the likelihood of its use during intercourse, but not increase frequency of sexual activity [6]. Given that more than 30 % of young women do not use a condom at the time of first intercourse, having this discussion prior to sexual debut is crucial.

ADOLESCENT AND YOUNG WOMEN AND DUAL-METHOD USE

Condoms, both male and female, are unique contraceptive options in that they are the only methods that protect against STIs, including HIV [1, 24]. However, they are not highly effective methods of preventing pregnancy [1, 17]. In the well-intended mission of preventing unintended pregnancies among teenaged women, many providers fail to discuss the additional benefits of condoms and instead focus on highly effective contraceptive methods.

A significant reduction in transmission of bacterial and parasitic STIs (such as chlamydia, gonorrhea, and trichomoniasis) provided by latex condoms is well documented [14]. However, specific data on the amount of risk reduction vary widely, from as much as 26 to 86 % [34, 35]. Latex condoms are also effective at decreasing transmission of sexually transmitted viruses. HPV transmission may decrease by as much as 70 % in couples who use condoms 100 %

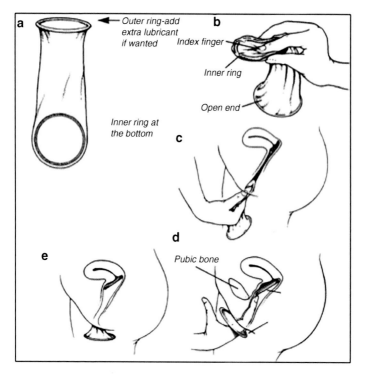

a Outer ring-add extra lubricant if wanted **b**

Index finger

Inner ring

Open end

Inner ring at the bottom **c**

d Pubic bone

e

Fig. 5.1 (**a**) Reality female condom. (**b**) Holding it for insertion. (**c**) Insertion. (**d**) Pushing the internal ring beyond the pubic bone, close to the uterine cervix, and (**e**) the device in place (From Kiley and Sobrero [55], with permission).

of the time and by as much as 50 % in couples who use condoms "most" of the time, compared to couples who use condoms less than 5 % of the time [36]. HIV transmission is reduced by about 80 % [37] and herpes simplex virus by about 30 % with consistent use [38, 39].

Lambskin condoms are less effective at preventing transmission of HIV, but condoms made from polyurethane appear to be as effective as latex condoms [40]. Female condoms also appear to be equally effective as male condoms at preventing other STI transmission [22, 41]. Some evidence also suggests that non-latex condoms may also decrease transmission of human papillomavirus [36] which is a major contributing cause of cervical cancer.

In addition to offering protection from infections, dual-method use offers additional contraceptive benefits, which are particularly important for young women on user-dependent contraceptive methods (i.e., oral contraceptive pills, transdermal patch, vaginal ring, and depo-medroxyprogesterone) [42]. The effectiveness of these methods tends to be lower than long-acting methods (i.e., IUDs and implants), yet they are the most common non-barrier methods used by adolescent women [5]. It is well documented that condom use and contraceptive pill use are inversely related, such that condom use declines when pill use improves [43–45].

In the last nationwide survey of adolescent women, 20 % reported using a condom at last sex in addition to another method [5]. This number has improved over the past several decades; in 2001 only 7 % reported using condoms in addition to another method [46]. These rates vary by race and ethnicity—24 % of non-Hispanic white adolescent women report using dual methods at last sex, while only 14 % of white Hispanic adolescent women and 13 % of black non-Hispanic women report using dual methods at last sex.

Several factors may predict an adolescent woman's decision to use two methods. Condom use, regardless of other method use, decreases rapidly once a sexual relationship is established [28]. The notion of a "safe partner" has been well documented, and young women are less likely to protect themselves from STIs (and pregnancy) with partners who they feel are safe [43, 46–48]. Older adolescents are more likely to use dual methods than their younger counterparts [5], and women who express avoiding pregnancy as the most important motivator for contraceptive use are more likely to use two methods [49]. Adolescent women living in an urban population who express a concern about acquiring HIV, or who have had an STI already, are also more likely to use dual methods [50].

STIs can have long-lasting implications, particularly for an adolescent population, and the importance of encouraging dual-method use among that population cannot be understated. It is essential to address both pregnancy and STI prevention in each adolescent visit.

OTHER BARRIER METHODS
Diaphragm, Cervical Cap, Sponges, and Spermicides
The use of other barrier methods, including diaphragms, cervical caps, sponges, and spermicides, is poorly studied in adolescent populations. Epidemiologic information on these barrier methods is not collected specifically for teens, and their use is uncommon [2, 5]. This lack of data is largely due to other methods that are both more available and more efficacious.

Nonetheless, these methods are available, and it is plausible that a young woman might request one as contraception. We recommend that providers encourage a patient seeking one of these methods to consider a more effective method of contraception. That said, we include brief descriptions of efficacy, as well as how to use the devices—in general these methods are more effective than using nothing. It is important to tell patients that these methods do no protect from STIs, including HIV.

Diaphragm

The diaphragm is a rubber device that a woman puts into her vagina herself; it blocks sperm from entering the cervix. The device must be fitted by a healthcare professional; ill-fitting diaphragms can allow sperm to pass and cause failure of the device. Traditionally the recommendation has been to fill the dome of the diaphragm with spermicide, although there is no evidence to support this practice [51]. The diaphragm is placed so that the posterior edge is in the posterior fornix of the vagina and the anterior edge is behind the pubic bone. The device must be in place prior to intercourse and must remain in place for 6 h afterwards. With typical use, 16 % of women will experience a pregnancy within a year; with perfect use, only 6 % will experience a pregnancy [24]. It is important to note that these statistics are generated from adult women and therefore may not represent efficacy rates in adolescent women.

Cervical Cap

The cervical cap is similar to the diaphragm, although it has a smaller diameter and is fit to cover the cervix completely. It also functions to block sperm and comes in several sizes that must be fitted by a healthcare provider. Efficacy rates vary by parity, and all are studies from adults rather than teens; with typical use 32 % of parous women will experience a pregnancy, while 16 % of nulliparous women will experience a pregnancy. Perfect use rates are slightly better, with 20 % of parous women and 9 % of nulliparous women experiencing a device failure. A Cochrane Database Review found that the cervical cap has similar efficacy rates to the diaphragm, although these rates may vary slightly by brand [52]. The cervical cap must be left in place for 8 h after intercourse and may be left in place for up to 2 days after placement. Women using the cervical cap must be able to accurately identify their own cervix to apply the device [17].

Vaginal Sponge

The contraceptive sponge is an over-the-counter product. It is a small, soft device filled with nonoxynl-9 spermicide. The device must be moistened with water and inserted deep into the vagina prior to intercourse. The sponge must be left in place for 6 h after intercourse and can remain in place for up to 24 h. Once the sponge is removed, it must be discarded. The sponge has among the highest failure rates of barrier contraception [53]— for parous women, typical-use failure rates approach 32 %, and for nulliparous women, the failure rate is 16 %. Perfect use failure rates are 20 % and 9 % for parous and nulliparous women, respectively [24].

Spermicides

Spermicides come in numerous delivery systems, including creams, gels, and suppositories. Efficacy rates are extremely broad, ranging from 5 to 50 % [54]. Some data suggests that they are no more effective than timed coitus [17]. Trials investigating spermicides as contraceptive options are also plagued by high attrition rates and difficulty with enrollment, both of which threaten the validity of most spermicide trials [54].

CONCLUSIONS

Condoms are the only method of contraception that prevents both STIs and pregnancy; however, they are far less effective at preventing pregnancy than hormonal and LARC methods. They are the most widely used method among adolescents, but are often used inconsistently and incorrectly; thus, the pregnancy rate and STI rate among condom users remain high. Condoms are most effective when utilized as part of a dual-method strategy, and contraception counseling for teens should focus on condom use as adjunct to more effective methods and as a necessity in STI prevention.

REFERENCES

1. Warner L, Steiner MJ. Male condoms. In: Hatcher RA, Trussell J, Nelson AL, et al, editor. Contraceptive technology. New York, NY: Ardent Media; 2008. p. 297–316.
2. Trends in sexual risk behaviors among high school students–United States, 1991–2001. MMWR Morb Mortal Wkly Rep. 2002;51(38):856–9.
3. Centers for Disease Control and Prevention. U.S. medical eligibility criteria for contraceptive use, 2010. MMWR. 2010;59(RR-4):1–86.
4. Reece M, Herbenick D, Schick V, Sanders SA, Dodge B, Fortenberry JD. Condom use rates in a national probability sample of males and females ages 14 to 94 in the United States. J Sex Med. 2010;7 Suppl 5:266–76.

5. Martinez G, Copen CE, Abma JC. Teenagers in the United States: sexual activity, contraceptive use, and childbearing, 2006–2010 national survey of family growth. Vital and health statistics series 23, data from the National Survey of Family. Growth. 2011;31:1–35.
6. Williams RL, Fortenberry JD. Update on adolescent condom use. Curr Opin Obstet Gynecol. 2011;23(5):350–4.
7. O'Sullivan LF, Udell W, Montrose VA, Antoniello P, Hoffman S. A cognitive analysis of college students' explanations for engaging in unprotected sexual intercourse. Arch Sex Behav. 2010;39(5): 1121–31.
8. Conard LA, Fortenberry JD, Blythe MJ, Orr DP. Pharmacists' attitudes toward and practices with adolescents. Arch Pediatr Adolesc Med. 2003;157(4):361–5.
9. Hoffman S, Mantell J, Exner T, Stein Z. The future of the female condom. Perspect Sex Reprod Health. 2004;36(3):120–6.
10. Eaton DK, Kann L, Kinchen S, Shanklin S, Ross J, Hawkins J, et al. Youth risk behavior surveillance–United States, 2007. MMWR Surveill Summ. 2008;57(4):1–131.
11. Kulczycki A, Kim DJ, Duerr A, Jamieson DJ, Macaluso M. The acceptability of the female and male condom: a randomized crossover trial. Perspect Sex Reprod Health. 2004;36(3):114–9.
12. McCabe E, Golub S, Lee AC. Making the female condom a "reality" for adolescents. J Pediatr Adolesc Gynecol. 1997;10(3):115–23.
13. Haignere CS, Gold R, Maskovsky J, Ambrosini J, Rogers CL, Gollub E. High-risk adolescents and female condoms: knowledge, attitudes, and use patterns. J Adolesc Health. 2000;26(6):392–8.
14. Stone KM, Grimes DA, Magder LS. Primary prevention of sexually transmitted diseases. A primer for clinicians. JAMA. 1986; 255(13):1763–6.
15. Van de Perre P, Jacobs D, Sprecher-Goldberger S. The latex condom, an efficient barrier against sexual transmission of AIDS-related viruses. AIDS. 1987;1(1):49–52.
16. Macaluso M, Lawson ML, Hortin G, Duerr A, Hammond KR, Blackwell R, et al. Efficacy of the female condom as a barrier to semen during intercourse. Am J Epidemiol. 2003;157(4):289–97.
17. Speroff L, Darney PD. Barrier methods of contraception. A clinical guide for contraception. Philadelphia, PA: Lippincott Williams & Wilkins; 2011.
18. Rosenberg MJ, Waugh MS. Latex condom breakage and slippage in a controlled clinical trial. Contraception. 1997;56(1):17–21.
19. Crosby R, Sanders S, Yarber WL, Graham CA. Condom-use errors and problems: a neglected aspect of studies assessing condom effectiveness. Am J Prev Med. 2003;24(4):367–70.
20. Steiner MJ, Dominik R, Rountree RW, Nanda K, Dorflinger LJ. Contraceptive effectiveness of a polyurethane condom and a latex condom: a randomized controlled trial. Obstet Gynecol. 2003;101(3):539–47.

21. Gallo MF, Grimes DA, Lopez LM, Schulz KF. Non-latex versus latex male condoms for contraception. Cochrane Database Syst Rev. 2006;(1):CD003550.
22. Macaluso M, Blackwell R, Jamieson DJ, Kulczycki A, Chen MP, Akers R, et al. Efficacy of the male latex condom and of the female polyurethane condom as barriers to semen during intercourse: a randomized clinical trial. Am J Epidemiol. 2007;166(1):88–96.
23. Trussell J, Sturgen K, Strickler J, Dominik R. Comparative contraceptive efficacy of the female condom and other barrier methods. Fam Plann Perspect. 1994;26(2):66–72.
24. Cates W, Raymond E. Vaginal barriers and spermicides. In: Hatcher RA, Ttussell J, Nelson AL, et al., editors. Contraceptive technology. New York, NY: Ardent Media; 2008.
25. Fihn SD, Boyko EJ, Chen CL, Normand EH, Yarbro P, Scholes D. Use of spermicide-coated condoms and other risk factors for urinary tract infection caused by Staphylococcus saprophyticus. Arch Intern Med. 1998;158(3):281–7.
26. Fihn SD, Boyko EJ, Normand EH, Chen CL, Grafton JR, Hunt M, et al. Association between use of spermicide-coated condoms and Escherichia coli urinary tract infection in young women. Am J Epidemiol. 1996;144(5):512–20.
27. Handley MA, Reingold AL, Shiboski S, Padian NS. Incidence of acute urinary tract infection in young women and use of male condoms with and without nonoxynol-9 spermicides. Epidemiology. 2002;13(4):431–6.
28. Fortenberry JD, Schick V, Herbenick D, Sanders SA, Dodge B, Reece M. Sexual behaviors and condom use at last vaginal intercourse: a national sample of adolescents ages 14 to 17 years. J Sex Med. 2010;7 Suppl 5:305–14.
29. Hamann CP, Kick SA. Update: immediate and delayed hypersensitivity to natural rubber latex. Cutis. 1993;52(5):307–11.
30. Chen FC, Buscher U, Niggemann B. Condoms are not a risk factor for sensitization to latex. Contraception. 2002;66(6):439–41.
31. Henry-Reid LM, O'Connor KG, Klein JD, Cooper E, Flynn P, Futterman DC. Current pediatrician practices in identifying high-risk behaviors of adolescents. Pediatrics. 2010;125(4):e741–7.
32. Martinez G, Abma J, Copen C. Educating teenagers about sex in the United States. NCHS Data Brief. 2010;44:1–8.
33. Jones RK, Purcell A, Singh S, Finer LB. Adolescents' reports of parental knowledge of adolescents' use of sexual health services and their reactions to mandated parental notification for prescription contraception. JAMA. 2005;293(3):340–8.
34. Holmes KK, Levine R, Weaver M. Effectiveness of condoms in preventing sexually transmitted infections. Bull World Health Organ. 2004;82(6):454–61.
35. Warner L, Stone KM, Macaluso M, Buehler JW, Austin HD. Condom use and risk of gonorrhea and Chlamydia: a systematic review of design and measurement factors assessed in epidemiologic studies. Sex Transm Dis. 2006;33(1):36–51.

36. Winer RL, Hughes JP, Feng Q, O'Reilly S, Kiviat NB, Holmes KK, et al. Condom use and the risk of genital human papillomavirus infection in young women. N Engl J Med. 2006;354(25):2645–54.
37. Weller S, Davis K. Condom effectiveness in reducing heterosexual HIV transmission. Cochrane Database Syst Rev. 2002;(1):CD003255.
38. Martin ET, Krantz E, Gottlieb SL, Magaret AS, Langenberg A, Stanberry L, et al. A pooled analysis of the effect of condoms in preventing HSV-2 acquisition. Arch Intern Med. 2009;169(13):1233–40.
39. Stanaway JD, Wald A, Martin ET, Gottlieb SL, Magaret AS. Case-crossover analysis of condom use and herpes simplex virus type 2 acquisition. Sex Transm Dis. 2012;39(5):388–93.
40. Rosenberg MJ, Waugh MS, Solomon HM, Lyszkowski AD. The male polyurethane condom: a review of current knowledge. Contraception. 1996;53(3):141–6.
41. Vijayakumar G, Mabude Z, Smit J, Beksinska M, Lurie M. A review of female-condom effectiveness: patterns of use and impact on protected sex acts and STI incidence. Int J STD AIDS. 2006;17(10):652–9.
42. Pazol K, Kramer MR, Hogue CJ. Condoms for dual protection: patterns of use with highly effective contraceptive methods. Public Health Rep. 2010;125(2):208–17.
43. Ott MA, Adler NE, Millstein SG, Tschann JM, Ellen JM. The trade-off between hormonal contraceptives and condoms among adolescents. Perspect Sex Reprod Health. 2002;34(1):6–14.
44. Roye CF. Condom use by Hispanic and African-American adolescent girls who use hormonal contraception. J Adolesc Health. 1998;23(4):205–11.
45. Santelli JS, Warren CW, Lowry R, Sogolow E, Collins J, Kann L, et al. The use of condoms with other contraceptive methods among young men and women. Fam Plann Perspect. 1997;29(6):261–7.
46. Anderson JE, Santelli J, Gilbert BC. Adolescent dual use of condoms and hormonal contraception: trends and correlates 1991–2001. Sex Transm Dis. 2003;30(9):719–22.
47. Brown JL, Hennessy M, Sales JM, DiClemente RJ, Salazar LF, Vanable PA, et al. Multiple method contraception use among African American adolescents in four US cities. Infect Dis Obstet Gynecol. 2011;2011:765917.
48. Manning WD, Longmore MA, Giordano PC. The relationship context of contraceptive use at first intercourse. Fam Plann Perspect. 2000;32(3):104–10.
49. Crosby RA, DiClemente RJ, Wingood GM, Sionean C, Cobb BK, Harrington K, et al. Correlates of using dual methods for sexually transmitted diseases and pregnancy prevention among high-risk African-American female teens. J Adolesc Health. 2001;28(5):410–4.
50. Riehman KS, Sly DF, Soler H, Eberstein IW, Quadagno D, Harrison DF. Dual-method use among an ethnically diverse group of women at risk of HIV infection. Fam Plann Perspect. 1998;30(5):212–7.

51. Cook L, Nanda K, Grimes D. Diaphragm versus diaphragm with spermicides for contraception. Cochrane Database Syst Rev. 2002;(3):CD002031.
52. Gallo MF, Grimes DA, Schulz KF. Cervical cap versus diaphragm for contraception. Cochrane Database Syst Rev. 2002;(4):CD003551.
53. Kuyoh MA, Toroitich-Ruto C, Grimes DA, Schulz KF, Gallo MF. Sponge versus diaphragm for contraception: a Cochrane review. Contraception. 2003;67(1):15–8.
54. Grimes DA, Lopez L, Raymond EG, Halpern V, Nanda K, Schulz KF. Spermicide used alone for contraception. Cochrane Database Syst Rev. 2005;(4):CD005218.
55. Kiley J, Sobrero A. Use and effectiveness of barrier and spermicidal contraceptive methods. The Global Library of Women's Medicine (ISSN: 1756–2228) 2008. doi:10.3843/GLOWM.10385.

Chapter 6
Emergency Contraception

Rachel B. Rapkin and Eleanor Bimla Schwarz

BACKGROUND
Unlike traditional methods of contraception that require advance planning, emergency contraception (EC) can be used *after* unprotected intercourse to prevent pregnancy. Although sometimes referred to as the "morning after pill," EC can be used up to 5 days after a contraceptive emergency.

Early Forms of EC
The first reported use of postcoital contraception was in the 1960s as a treatment for rape victims [1]. In 1974, Yuzpe and colleagues published their findings on the use of combined oral contraceptives for postcoital contraception [2]. At the same time, Kesseru and colleagues evaluated progestin-only EC regimens [3]. In 1998, the US Food and Drug Administration (FDA) approved Preven™, a two-dose regimen that contained a total of ethinyl estradiol (EE) 20 µg with levonorgestrel (LNG) 100 µg divided among four pills [4].

R.B. Rapkin, M.D., M.P.H. (✉)
Department of Obstetrics and Gynecology, University of South Florida,
2 Tampa General Circle, 6th Floor, Tampa, FL 33606, USA
e-mail: rrapkin@health.usf.edu

E.B. Schwarz, M.D., M.S.
Women's Health Services Research Unit, Center for Research on Health Care, University of Pittsburgh, 230 McKee Place Suite 600, Pittsburgh, PA 15213, USA

A. Whitaker and M. Gilliam (eds.), *Contraception for Adolescent and Young Adult Women*, DOI 10.1007/978-1-4614-6579-9_6,
© Springer Science+Business Media New York 2014

The Copper Intrauterine Device
Although using an IUD for EC was described as early as 1976, many US clinicians remain unaware of this option [5]. The copper intrauterine device (Cu-IUD) is the most effective method of emergency contraception, yet it is currently the least utilized. In addition to being over 99 % effective at preventing pregnancy when inserted as EC, it can continue to provide long-term, reversible contraception for up to 10 years or more [6].

Levonorgestrel-Only EC
A LNG-only method of EC containing two 0.75 mg LNG tablets known as Plan B® was FDA approved in 1999, after it was demonstrated to be more effective and have fewer side effects than Preven™ [7]. In 2009, the FDA approved Next Choice, a generic version of Plan B® and Plan B One-Step®, a single 1.5 mg LNG pill, which was shown to be as effective as the two-dose regimen [8]. In June 2013, after an unusually prolonged and political review and an extended court battle, the FDA approved Plan B One-Step use without a prescription and without age or point-of-sale restrictions.

Ulipristal Acetate EC
Ulipristal acetate (UPA) was FDA approved for use as EC up to 120 h after unprotected intercourse, under the brand name ella™ in 2010. The major benefit of UPA is its increased effectiveness compared to LNG, especially after more than 72 h since unprotected intercourse and for obese women [9].

UPA is a second-generation progesterone receptor modulator. Low doses of mifepristone, a first generation antiprogestin, was shown to be more effective and have fewer side effects than the Yuzpe regimen as early as 1991 [10–12]. Low-dose mifepristone is currently available for EC in Russia, China, and Vietnam. However, because higher doses of mifepristone can be used to induce abortion, women are not able to access mifepristone for EC in countries (including the United States) that restrict access to pregnancy termination services.

EPIDEMIOLOGY
Many US teens face a need for EC. At first intercourse, 22 % of teenagers report using *no* form of contraception [13]. Although the large majority of sexually experienced teenagers report having ever used some method of contraception, the methods most commonly used by US teens are those with the highest risks of failure: condoms, withdrawal, and oral contraceptives [13]. Over the last decade, ever use of EC by all US women of reproductive

age has increased from 4 % in 2002 to 10 % in 2006–2008; ever use among US teenagers increased from 8 % in 2002 to 14 % in 2006–2010 [13, 14].

MECHANISM OF ACTION
The three available methods of EC (the copper IUD, UPA, and LNG) each have different mechanisms of action and will be reviewed separately.

The Copper Intrauterine Device
The mechanism of action of the Cu-IUD remains an area of active inquiry. Existing studies indicate that the IUD creates a "foreign body effect" resulting in a sterile inflammatory reaction that is toxic to sperm and ova. The increase in copper ions affects enzymes, prostaglandins, and white blood cells that impair sperm function [15, 16] and may prevent implantation of a fertilized embryo [17, 18].

Levonorgestrel-Only EC
Levonorgestrel EC, like many other hormonal contraceptives, prevents pregnancy primarily by delaying or inhibiting ovulation and inhibiting fertilization. When given prior to the rise in luteinizing hormone (LH), LNG inhibits or delays and blunts the LH peak, delaying or preventing follicular development [19, 20]. Studies demonstrate that when used as EC, LNG has no effect on the endometrium and therefore does not work by preventing the implantation of a fertilized embryo. It is not an abortifacient [21]. In vitro studies do not demonstrate a direct effect of LNG on sperm function [3]. When used as a daily contraceptive, a primary mechanism of action of LNG is to thicken cervical mucus. However, this is not likely LNG's primary mechanism of action when used as EC.

Ulipristal Acetate EC
Similar to LNG, UPA inhibits follicular rupture when given prior to the LH rise. However, UPA also delays ovulation when taken on the day of the LH peak [22]. Unlike LNG EC, one study found that UPA alters the endometrium. It is not known whether this may inhibit implantation [23].

CONTRACEPTIVE EFFICACY AND EFFECTIVENESS
To determine the effectiveness of EC, one must first calculate the number of pregnancies that would be expected to occur in the absence of EC. This is estimated by using published data on the probability of pregnancy during each day of the menstrual cycle

but is difficult because women rarely precisely recall the details of their menstrual cycles, precluding accurate assessment of fertile days [24, 25]. This has resulted in recent concerns that some may have initially *overestimated* the efficacy of EC [24]. However, it is clear that pregnancy rates after use of LNG or UPA EC are lower than after using the Yuzpe regimen and lower than after using no method of contraception [26].

The Copper Intrauterine Device

Multiple trials have evaluated the effectiveness of the Cu-IUD for EC. Combined, these trials report a total of three pregnancies in 3,470 women, demonstrating a pregnancy rate of 0.09 %, making the Cu-IUD the most effective method of emergency contraception [12]. Study of the use of the LNG-IUD for EC is ongoing, but as of now, there is no evidence that it is effective for emergency contraception.

Levonorgestrel-Only EC

Plan B® was approved on the basis of a double-blind randomized trial conducted by the WHO which demonstrated an almost three-fold higher incidence of pregnancy among women who used the Yuzpe regimen compared to those who used the LNG regimen [7]. It was estimated that LNG prevented 95 % of expected pregnancies when taken within 24 hours of unprotected intercourse; pregnancy rates decreased by 85 % when taken 25–48 and by 58 % when taken 49–72 hours following unprotected intercourse. A reevaluation of the WHO study and a second large study comparing the Yuzpe regimen to LNG calculated that at least 49 % of pregnancies expected under the Yuzpe regimen would be prevented using LNG [26]. Thus, even if the Yuzpe regimen does not prevent *any* pregnancies, LNG has an efficacy rate of 49 %. Because the Yuzpe method *has* been shown to prevent or delay ovulation, it likely has at least some effect in preventing pregnancy, and therefore LNG EC is *at least* 49 % effective [26].

Ulipristal Acetate EC

One large prospective study followed women who took UPA EC up to 120 h after intercourse. By comparing the number of observed pregnancies to the number expected, the authors estimate that UPA EC is 62 % effective [27]. In addition, two large randomized trials have compared the efficacy of UPA and LNG for EC [28, 29]. Both found UPA to be at least as effective as LNG in preventing pregnancy when taken within 72 hours after unprotected intercourse. Importantly, unlike what has been seen with LNG, the efficacy of UPA does not appear to decline when taken up to 48–72 h after unprotected intercourse. A meta-analysis of these studies demonstrated that women's risk of pregnancy after taking UPA was almost half that of women who took LNG within 120 h after intercourse [29].

Factors Affecting EC Effectiveness

Several factors increase the chances that a woman will become pregnant despite use of EC. These include repeated acts of unprotected intercourse, a contraceptive emergency close to ovulation, and obesity [9]. Compared to normal or underweight women, obese women face up to four times the risk of pregnancy after using LNG and twice the risk of pregnancy after using UPA. Thus, obese women and teens should be particularly encouraged to consider using a Cu-IUD or UPA instead of LNG EC.

Studies Showing Better or Worse Effectiveness Among Young Women

Studies of the use of EC by teens as young as 11 years of age have shown that teens are as able as older women to identify the need for EC and safely and effectively use EC [30]. Because teens are generally more fertile than older women, the failure rates of all contraceptives may be higher than those commonly quoted [31].

SIDE EFFECTS

Headache, Nausea, and Vomiting

The most common side effects with LNG and UPA EC include headache (4–19 %), nausea (3–23 %), dysmenorrhea (4–14 %), fatigue (3–17 %), abdominal pain (4–18 %), and dizziness (3–10 %) [7, 8, 27–29]. The incidence of vomiting reported with these methods is very low at only 2 % [28]. This is in stark contrast to the Yuzpe method, which caused nausea and vomiting in 50 % and 20 % of women, respectively [7, 32]. Table 6.1 contains a summary of the most commonly experienced side effects after using oral EC.

Menstrual Changes

Women experience variable changes in their menses after taking EC. Some women report a reduction in cycle length, while others report an increase in cycle length of up to 2 weeks [27, 28]. On average, women experience their next menses within 3 weeks of taking EC; those who do not should be tested for pregnancy. Women who take UPA may also report intermenstrual bleeding, most commonly described as spotting [27].

TABLE 6.1 Percentage of patients who experience side effects with oral emergency contraception.

Side effect	UPA [27–29]	LNG [7, 8, 28, 29]	Yuzpe method [7, 32]
Headache	4–19	4–19	20
Nausea	4–13	3–23	51
Dysmenorrhea	4–13	14	n/a[a]
Fatigue	3–6	4–17	29
Abdominal pain	4–7	4–18	21
Dizziness	3–5	2–11	17
Vomiting	<1	<1–1	19
Diarrhea	2	1–4	n/a[a]
Change in cycle length (days)	+2.6	–2.1	n/a[a]

[a]Data not available

Copper IUD Side Effects

The side effects women experience while using the Cu-IUD for EC are similar to those experienced when the Cu-IUD is used for ongoing contraception. (See Chap. 2—Intrauterine Devices.) The most common side effects include cramping and bleeding irregularities. IUDs do not increase teens' risk of thromboembolism, acquiring sexually transmitted infections (STIs), pelvic inflammatory disease, or infertility. Because of their superior safety and effectiveness, the American College of Obstetricians and Gynecologists recommends that all women and adolescents consider IUDs as first-line contraceptives [33–35].

Effects of EC on Exposed Pregnancies

Pregnancies that occur with a copper IUD in place have an increased risk of spontaneous abortion but have resulted in healthy births [36]. Women who become pregnant despite using LNG EC, or who inadvertently take LNG EC after conception has occurred, do not appear to face an increased risk of miscarriage, congenital malformations, perinatal complications, or any other adverse pregnancy outcomes [37]. Although there have been several case reports of ectopic pregnancies following LNG EC, a systematic review found that women who use LNG EC are not at increased risk of ectopic pregnancy compared to the general population [38–41]. Because EC decreases the overall risk of pregnancy, the risk of ectopic pregnancy is likewise reduced. There are currently no published studies reporting the outcomes of pregnancies exposed to UPA.

CONTINUATION AND FOLLOW-UP
No follow-up is routinely required after using EC. According to the Centers for Disease Control and Prevention and the US Preventive Services Task Force, females aged ≤ 25 years should be screened annually for chlamydia and gonorrhea, although this testing should not delay provision of EC [42, 43]. When possible, health-care providers should discuss the factors that placed the adolescent at risk for unintended pregnancy and review available methods of contraception to reduce future risk of facing a similar contraceptive emergency. However, these conversations should not delay access to or provision of EC. Teens should be instructed to seek pregnancy testing if they have not experienced menses within 3 weeks of using EC.

While the Cu-IUD can provide teens with both highly effective emergency and ongoing contraception, women who repeatedly use oral EC face higher rates of unintended pregnancy than those using other contraceptives and should be encouraged to start a continuous method of contraception after use of EC. The US Selected Practice Recommendations (SPR) for Contraceptive Use state that any regular contraceptive method can be started immediately after use of oral EC but that a barrier method (or abstinence) should be used for 14 days after UPA and 7 days after LNG EC use. If a woman does not have a withdrawal bleed within 3 weeks, the SPR recommends obtaining a pregnancy test [44]. Other than unintended pregnancy, there are no known health risks related to repeated use of EC. The label for ella™ states that "repeated use of ella within the same menstrual cycle is not recommended, as safety and efficacy of repeat use within the same cycle has not been evaluated" [45]. Clinicians should be aware that teens who repeatedly seek EC may be more likely to be experiencing sexual or reproductive coercion; thus, screening for coercion, as well as provision on information on healthy relationships, and local resources can be helpful [46].

ISSUES FOR ADOLESCENTS AND YOUNG WOMEN
Prescription Requirement for Teenagers
There is no medical reason to obtain a prescription prior to obtaining EC, but this requirement persisted for many years after EC was first approved by the FDA and posed a major barrier to adolescents' obtaining EC in a timely fashion, potentially compromising its efficacy [47]. Several medical organizations, including the American College of Obstetricians and Gynecologists, the American Academy of Pediatrics, and the Society for Adolescent Medicine, recommended making EC available over the counter to

individuals of all ages [48–50]. As of June 2013, after many iterations of age and point-of-sale restrictions, extended FDA review, and court involvement, the FDA approved Plan B One-Step for use without a prescription and without age or point-of-sale restrictions. UPA EC continues to require a prescription for use.

Pharmacy Access and Advance Provision for Adolescents
One concern with advance provision of and unrestricted access to EC has been that it may increase risky sexual behavior. However, in a study that randomized teens to pharmacy access, advance provision, or standard clinic access, teens who received advance provision of EC were found to use EC more frequently, yet had the same incidence of STIs as women in the other two groups [51]. Similarly, a number of other studies have evaluated the effect of advance provision of EC and consistently found that advance provision increases timely use of EC [52–56].

Discussing EC with Teens
Teens may have limited or incorrect knowledge of EC; thus, clinicians should routinely provide information about all postcoital options [50, 57]. Counseling should include a description of the safety and relative effectiveness of all available methods of EC. When a prescription is required, teens should be encouraged to fill a prescription in advance of need to facilitate prompt use when needed.

REFERENCES
1. Morris JM, Van Wagenen G. Compounds interfering with ovum implantation and development 3. The role of estrogens. Am J Obstet Gynecol. 1966;96(6):804–15.
2. Yuzpe AA, Thurlow HJ, Ramzy I, Leyshon JI. Post coital contraception—a pilot study. J Reprod Med. 1974;13(2):53–8.
3. Kesseru E, Garmendia F, Westphal N, Parada J. The hormonal and peripheral effects of d-norgestrel in postcoital contraception. Contraception. 1974;10(4):411–24.
4. First emergency contraceptive product hits U.S. market shelves. Contracept Technol Update. 1998;19(11):141–3.
5. Lippes J, Malik T, Tatum HJ. The postcoital copper-T. Adv Plan Parent. 1976;11(1):24–9.
6. Long-term reversible contraception. Twelve years of experience with the TCu380A and TCu220C. Contraception. 1997;56(6):341–52.
7. Randomised controlled trial of levonorgestrel versus the Yuzpe regimen of combined oral contraceptives for emergency contraception. Task Force on Postovulatory Methods of Fertility Regulation. Lancet. 1998;352(9126):428–33.

8. von Hertzen H, Piaggio G, Ding J, Chen J, Song S, Bartfai G, et al. Low dose mifepristone and two regimens of levonorgestrel for emergency contraception: a WHO multicentre randomised trial. Lancet. 2002;360(9348):1803–10.
9. Glasier A, Cameron ST, Blithe D, Scherrer B, Mathe H, Levy D, et al. Can we identify women at risk of pregnancy despite using emergency contraception? Data from randomized trials of ulipristal acetate and levonorgestrel. Contraception. 2011;84(4):363–7.
10. Glasier A, Thong KJ, Dewar M, Mackie M, Baird DT. Postcoital contraception with mifepristone. Lancet. 1991;337(8754):1414–5.
11. Webb AM. Alternative treatments in oral postcoital contraception: interim results. Adv Contracept. 1991;7(2–3):271–9.
12. Cheng L, Gulmezoglu AM, Piaggio G, Ezcurra E, Van Look PF. Interventions for emergency contraception. Cochrane Database Syst Rev. 2008;(2):CD001324.
13. Martinez G, Copen CE, Abma JC. Teenagers in the United States: sexual activity, contraceptive use, and childbearing, 2006–2010 national survey of family growth. Vital Health Stat 23. 2011;31:1–35.
14. Mosher WD, Jones J. Use of contraception in the United States: 1982–2008. Vital Health Stat 23. 2010;29:1–44.
15. Sagiroglu N. Phagocytosis of spermatozoa in the uterine cavity of woman using intrauterine device. Int J Fertil. 1971;16(1):1–14.
16. Ammala M, Nyman T, Strengell L, Rutanen EM. Effect of intrauterine contraceptive devices on cytokine messenger ribonucleic acid expression in the human endometrium. Fertil Steril. 1995;63(4):773–8.
17. El-Habashi M, El-Sahwi S, Gawish S, Osman M. Effect of Lippes loop on sperm recovery from human fallopian tubes. Contraception. 1980;22(5):549–55.
18. Ortiz ME, Croxatto HB, Bardin CW. Mechanisms of action of intrauterine devices. Obstet Gynecol Surv. 1996;51(12 Suppl):S42–51.
19. Hapangama D, Glasier AF, Baird DT. The effects of peri-ovulatory administration of levonorgestrel on the menstrual cycle. Contraception. 2001;63(3):123–9.
20. Marions L, Cekan SZ, Bygdeman M, Gemzell-Danielsson K. Effect of emergency contraception with levonorgestrel or mifepristone on ovarian function. Contraception. 2004;69(5):373–7.
21. Durand M, del Carmen Cravioto M, Raymond EG, et al. The mechanism of action of short-term levonorgestrel administration in emergency contraception. Contraception. 2001;64:227–34.
22. Brache V, Cochon L, Jesam C, Maldonado R, Salvatierra AM, Levy DP, et al. Immediate pre-ovulatory administration of 30 mg ulipristal acetate significantly delays follicular rupture. Hum Reprod. 2010;25(9):2256–63.
23. Stratton P, Levens ED, Hartog B, Piquion J, Wei Q, Merino M, et al. Endometrial effects of a single early luteal dose of the selective progesterone receptor modulator CDB-2914. Fertil Steril. 2010;93(6):2035–41.

24. Trussell J, Ellertson C, von Hertzen H, Bigrigg A, Webb A, Evans M, et al. Estimating the effectiveness of emergency contraceptive pills. Contraception. 2003;67(4):259–65.
25. Stirling A, Glasier A. Estimating the efficacy of emergency contraception—how reliable are the data? Contraception. 2002;66(1):19–22.
26. Raymond E, Taylor D, Trussell J, Steiner MJ. Minimum effectiveness of the levonorgestrel regimen of emergency contraception. Contraception. 2004;69(1):79–81.
27. Fine P, Mathe H, Ginde S, Cullins V, Morfesis J, Gainer E. Ulipristal acetate taken 48–120 hours after intercourse for emergency contraception. Obstet Gynecol. 2010;115(2 Pt 1):257–63.
28. Creinin MD, Schlaff W, Archer DF, Wan L, Frezieres R, Thomas M, et al. Progesterone receptor modulator for emergency contraception: a randomized controlled trial. Obstet Gynecol. 2006;108(5): 1089–97.
29. Glasier AF, Cameron ST, Fine PM, Logan SJ, Casale W, Van Horn J, et al. Ulipristal acetate versus levonorgestrel for emergency contraception: a randomised non-inferiority trial and meta-analysis. Lancet. 2010;375(9714):555–62.
30. Raine TR, Ricciotti N, Sokoloff A, Brown BA, Hummel A, Harper CC. An over-the-counter simulation study of a single-tablet emergency contraceptive in young females. Obstet Gynecol. 2012; 119(4):772–9.
31. Teal SB, Sheeder J. IUD use in adolescent mothers: retention, failure and reasons for discontinuation. Contraception. 2012;85(3): 270–4.
32. Ho PC, Kwan MS. A prospective randomized comparison of levonorgestrel with the Yuzpe regimen in post-coital contraception. Hum Reprod. 1993;8(3):389–92.
33. Committee ACOG. Opinion no. 450: Increasing use of contraceptive implants and intrauterine devices to reduce unintended pregnancy. Obstet Gynecol. 2009;114(6):1434–8.
34. Committee on Adolescent Health Care Long-Acting Reversible Contraception Working Group, The American College of Obstetricians and Gynecologists. Committee opinion no. 539: adolescents and long-acting reversible contraception: implants and intrauterine devices. Obstet Gynecol. 2012;120:983–8.
35. American College of Obstetricians and Gynecologists. ACOG Practice Bulletin No. 121: long-acting reversible contraception: implants and intrauterine devices. Obstet Gynecol. 2011;118(1): 184–96.
36. Brahmi D, Steenland MW, Renner RM, Gaffield ME, Curtis KM. Pregnancy outcomes with an IUD in situ: a systematic review. Contraception. 2012;85(2):131–9.
37. Zhang L, Chen J, Wang Y, Ren F, Yu W, Cheng L. Pregnancy outcome after levonorgestrel-only emergency contraception failure: a prospective cohort study. Hum Reprod. 2009;24(7):1605–11.

38. Ghosh B, Dadhwal V, Deka D, Ramesan CK, Mittal S. Ectopic pregnancy following levonorgestrel emergency contraception: a case report. Contraception. 2009;79(2):155–7.
39. Cabar FR, Pereira PP, Zugaib M. Ectopic pregnancy following levonorgestrel emergency contraception. Contraception. 2009;80(2):227; author reply 227–8.
40. Kozinszky Z, Bakken RT, Lieng M. Ectopic pregnancy after levonorgestrel emergency contraception. Contraception. 2011;83(3):281–3.
41. Cleland K, Raymond E, Trussell J, Cheng L, Zhu H. Ectopic pregnancy and emergency contraceptive pills: a systematic review. Obstet Gynecol. 2010;115(6):1263–6.
42. Workowski KA, Berman S. Sexually transmitted diseases treatment guidelines 2010. MMWR Recomm Rep. 2010;59(RR-12): 1–110.
43. U.S. Preventive Services Task Force. Screening for chlamydial infection: U.S. Preventive Services Task Force recommendation statement. Ann Intern Med. 2007;147(2):128–34.
44. Centers for Disease Control and Prevention. U.S. selected practice recommendations for contraceptive use, 2013. MMWR Recomm Rep. 2013;62(5):1–64.
45. ella [package insert]. Morristown, NJ: Watson Pharmaceuticals; 2010. http://www.accessdata.fda.gov/drugsatfda_docs/label/2010/022474s000lbl.pdf. Accessed 1 Apr 2012.
46. Miller E, Decker MR, Raj A, Reed E, Marable D, Silverman JG. Intimate partner violence and health care-seeking patterns among female users of urban adolescent clinics. Matern Child Health J. 2010;14(6):910–7.
47. Wilkinson TA, Fahey N, Suther E, Cabral HJ, Silverstein M. Access to emergency contraception for adolescents. JAMA. 2012;307(4): 362–3.
48. American College of Obstetricians and Gynecologists. ACOG Practice Bulletin No. 112: emergency contraception. Obstet Gynecol. 2010;115(5):1100–9.
49. American Academy of Pediatrics Committee on Adolescence. Emergency contraception. Pediatrics. 2005;116(4):1026–35.
50. Gold MA, Sucato GS, Conard LA, Hillard PJ. Provision of emergency contraception to adolescents. J Adolesc Health. 2004;35(1): 67–70.
51. Raine TR, Harper CC, Rocca CH, Fischer R, Padian N, Klausner JD, et al. Direct access to emergency contraception through pharmacies and effect on unintended pregnancy and STIs: a randomized controlled trial. JAMA. 2005;293(1):54–62.
52. Gold MA, Wolford JE, Smith KA, Parker AM. The effects of advance provision of emergency contraception on adolescent women's sexual and contraceptive behaviors. J Pediatr Adolesc Gynecol. 2004;17(2):87–96.

53. Belzer M, Sanchez K, Olson J, Jacobs AM, Tucker D. Advance supply of emergency contraception: a randomized trial in adolescent mothers. J Pediatr Adolesc Gynecol. 2005;18(5):347–54.
54. Raymond EG, Stewart F, Weaver M, Monteith C, Van Der Pol B. Impact of increased access to emergency contraceptive pills: a randomized controlled trial. Obstet Gynecol. 2006;108(5): 1098–106.
55. Harper CC, Cheong M, Rocca CH, Darney PD, Raine TR. The effect of increased access to emergency contraception among young adolescents. Obstet Gynecol. 2005;106(3):483–91.
56. Rocca CH, Schwarz EB, Stewart FH, Darney PD, Raine TR, Harper CC. Beyond access: acceptability, use and nonuse of emergency contraception among young women. Am J Obstet Gynecol. 2007;196(1):29.e1–6; discussion 90.e1–5.
57. Johnson R, Nshom M, Nye AM, Cohall AT. There's always Plan B: adolescent knowledge, attitudes and intention to use emergency contraception. Contraception. 2010;81(2):128–32.

Chapter 7
Emerging Methods and Methods Not Available in the United States

Ellie J. Birtley and Patricia A. Lohr

INTRODUCTION

This chapter aims to put contraception in an international context and provide a glimpse of potential changes in the contraceptive landscape. It highlights the differences in the availability of methods in other countries and acts as a reminder of what can be learned from their experiences. We group contraceptives by methods and describe the emerging methods and those not available in the United States. Each method is described briefly, its efficacy and acceptability outlined, and its particular relevance to adolescents discussed. Table 7.1 summarizes the methods reviewed in this chapter. Emerging methods were mainly restricted to those in phase III clinical trials.

INTRAUTERINE DEVICES
Copper-Releasing Intrauterine Devices

There are currently two types of intrauterine devices (IUDs) available in the United States: the copper T 380A (CuT380A, ParaGard®) and the levonorgestrel-releasing intrauterine system (LNG-IUS, Mirena®). Outside of the United States, there are a variety of

E.J. Birtley, B.M., M.F.S.R.H.
Solent NHS Trust, Sexual Health, St. Mary's Community Health Campus,
2nd Floor, Milton Rd, Portsmouth, PO3 6AD, UK
e-mail: ellie.birtley@solent.nhs.uk

P.A. Lohr, M.D., M.P.H. (✉)
British Pregnancy Advisory Service, 20 Timothy's Bridge Road,
Stratford Enterprise Park, Stratford Upon Avon, CV37 9BF, UK
e-mail: patricia.lohr@bpas.org

A. Whitaker and M. Gilliam (eds.), *Contraception for Adolescent and Young Adult Women*, DOI 10.1007/978-1-4614-6579-9_7,
© Springer Science + Business Media New York 2014

TABLE 7.1   Emerging contraceptive methods and those not available in the United States included in this chapter.

Contraceptive group	Methods not available in the United States	Emerging methods
Intrauterine devices	Mini TT 380® Slimline	Alternative/generic versions of Mirena®
	UT 380 Short®	
	Multisafe® 375 Short	
	GyneFix®	
	FibroPlant®	
	Femilis®	
	γ Cu380 IUD	
Combined hormonal contraception	Cyclofem®	Nestorone® and ethinyl estradiol contraceptive vaginal ring
	Mesigyna®	
	Deladroxate	
	Injectable No. 1	
Progestin-only contraception	Jadelle®	Ulipristal acetate vaginal ring
	Sino-implant (II)	
	Noristerat®	
	Cerazette®	
	Progering®	
Barrier methods	Female condom	Woman's Condom
	Cupid female condom	SILCS diaphragm
	VA w.o.w./V'Amour/Reddy	
	Phoenurse female condom	
	Panty Condom	

IUDs available providing a range of designs and sizes reflecting the belief that one size does not fit all. In 1980, Hasson creatively described this view by writing, "Individual variations in the size and shape of the human uterus are probably greater than variations in the size and shape of the human foot" [1].

Nulliparous women have smaller uterine dimensions than parous women [2, 3] and are also more likely to experience expulsion and early removal of copper IUDs for pain and bleeding [4]. Failed and difficult fittings also appear to occur more frequently in this group possibly due to differences in cervical canal

TABLE 7.2 Characteristics of selected small versions of framed copper-bearing IUDs compared with the standard Cu T380A.

Device	Copper surface area (mm²)	Width (mm)	Length (mm)	Loading tube width (mm)	Minimum uterine depth (cm)	Duration of use (years)
Mini TT 380® Slimline (banded)	380	23.2	29.5	4.75	5	5
UT 380 Short®	380	32	28	3.6	5–7	5
Multisafe® 375 Short	375	19.5	29.4	3.85	5–7	5
Cu T380A®	380	32	36	4.4	6.5	10

size [5]. Smaller-framed and frameless intrauterine contraceptives have been developed to accommodate differences in uterine and cervical size and thereby expand access [6].

Table 7.2 summarizes the characteristics of selected smaller-framed copper IUDs compared with the standard Cu T380A. There is limited evidence supporting the benefits of these IUDs over ones with a standard size frame. One unblinded randomized trial compared the Cu T380A to two devices designed for nulliparous women, the CuT380 Nul (designed for the study) and the u-shaped multiload Cu 375 short loop (ML Cu 375 sl) [7]. Continuation rates at 1 year for TCu 380 A, TCu 380 Nul, and ML Cu 375 sl were 29.5 %, 85.9 %, and 85.4 %, respectively ($p < 0.001$). Failure rates and removals for pain and bleeding were significantly lower in the women who received the smaller devices. The overall low continuation rate and high discontinuation rates for pain and bleeding associated with the CuT380A are inconsistent with other trials of this device in nulliparous women. These disparate findings suggest the effect of potential biases, for example, the study was unblinded [8]. While there is insufficient evidence that any particular framed copper device is better suited to younger or nulliparous women [9], the Faculty of Sexual and Reproductive Healthcare in the United Kingdom has advised that the smaller devices may be of use in women with uterine lengths of less than 6.5 cm when a standard device cannot be fitted [10].

Frameless devices include the GyneFix® 330 IUD which consists of six (standard version) or four copper sleeves (small version or GyneFix® 200) each 5 mm long and 2.2 mm in diameter, threaded on a length of polypropylene suture material [6]. Crimping of the upper and lower sleeves onto the suture prevents them from falling off. The proximal end of the thread is knotted which, at insertion, is anchored in the fundal myometrium with a specially designed inserter. The provider must acquire proficiency in the insertion technique, and the paucity of such trained inserters in the United Kingdom acts as a barrier to access.

The GyneFix® is highly efficacious, comparable to the TCu380A [11], but an increased rate of expulsion in the first year may limit the effectiveness of the frameless device. In a randomized trial, the first-year expulsion rate for the frameless IUD was 5.3 per 100 (95 % CI: 4.4–6.4) and 2.5 (95 % CI: 1.9–3.3) for the TCu380A [12]. The 8-year cumulative discontinuation rates for bleeding and/ or pain were the same for the two devices. This study also concluded that the 8-year discontinuation rates for pain alone were significantly lower for the frameless IUD ($p = 0.15$) but equivalent for bleeding or bleeding and pain ($p = 0.883$).

In addition to the smaller-framed or frameless devices, the Nova-T 380® IUD is available in the United Kingdom. The device has copper wire wound around a silver core but no copper banding on the arms allowing for a narrower loading tube width of 3.6 mm [13]. Compared with the 4.4 mm insertion tube of the TCu380A, some providers find the Nova-T 380® easier to insert in women with a narrow cervical os. The device is approved for 5 years of use and has been compared to the TCu380S [14]. When compared to the TCu380s, there were twice as many discontinuations of the Nova-T due to pregnancy in the first year of use; however, at 5 years, the rate difference was no longer significant at 2.3 % (95 % CI: 0.6–5.2) [14].

In Shanghai, a novel indomethacin-containing copper IUD aimed at reducing menstrual bleeding is manufactured [15]. The γ Cu380 IUD is composed of a gamma-shaped stainless steel frame with a spiral copper wire of 380 mm² in the middle layer. Two Silastic beads welded to the ends of the horizontal arms and a 26×26 mm Silastic ring placed in the middle of the device are loaded with a total of 25 mg indomethacin. A randomized clinical trial comparing the γ Cu380 IUD with the TCu380A demonstrated similar performance but lower rates of removal for bleeding with the indomethacin-treated device [16].

Levonorgestrel-Releasing Intrauterine Devices
The Mirena® intrauterine system releases 20 μg levonorgestrel daily for 5 years and is available worldwide offering highly effective, reversible contraception with a range of non-contraceptive health benefits. Alternative levonorgestrel-releasing devices have been

developed in Belgium by Wildemeersch and Rowe and a "slimline Mini-Mirena" has just become available in the United States [17].

The FibroPlant® is a frameless device that consists of a thread with a knot at its proximal end and a fibrous delivery system that is 1.6 mm wide and 3 cm long (FibroPlant 14) or 4.5 cm long (FibroPlant 20) and releases 14 or 20 µg of LNG per day, respectively [6]. In a non-comparative prospective trial, 304 women were fitted with a FibroPlant 20 and followed for 5 years (11,299 woman-months) [18]. The mean age of the cohort was 34.7 with a range of 15–48years and 14 % of the cohort was nulliparous. One pregnancy was observed following a silent expulsion giving a failure rate of 0.4 % (95 % CI: 0.0–1.06) in the first year of use. There were two expulsions and two perforations over 5 years (2.1 %, 95 % CI: 0.06–4.14) and a total discontinuation rate of 23.6 %, 95 % CI: 18.23–29.05. No comparative trials have been published.

The Femilis® is a small T-shaped levonorgestrel-containing device which lasts for 5 years [6]. The standard version is 28 mm wide and 30 mm long, with a drug delivery compartment on its stem releasing 20 µg LNG daily and an insertion width of 2.4 mm. The loading technique is simplified by the cross arm remaining outside the inserter tube. To compare, the Mirena® is 32 mm wide and 32 mm long with a loading tube width of 4.4 mm. In a prospective, non-comparative study, 288 insertions of Femilis® occurred and were followed up for 8,028 women-months [19]. Forty percent of the study population was nulliparous. Overall there were 9 removals for pain, 4 removals for bleeding problems, 14 for medical reasons, and 12 for nonmedical reasons. Femilis® was equally acceptable to nulliparous and parous women.

Uteron Pharma Operations and Medicines360 currently have a generic version of Mirena® in phase III clinical trial with the aim of gaining regulatory approval through the US Food and Drug Administration [20]. This product could be available at a lower price than Mirena®, thus increasing availability especially in countries where women pay the cost of the contraceptive.

COMBINED HORMONAL CONTRACEPTION
Combined Injectable Contraceptives

Combined injectable contraceptives (CICs) were introduced in the late 1980s and are available in Latin America, Asia, and Africa [21]. Like other combined hormonal methods, they contain an estrogen and a progestin and inhibit ovulation. Unlike progestin-only injectables, CICs are administered monthly and the fall in estradiol levels in the latter 2 weeks causes cyclic bleeding. Several formulations are available, and three of these have been compared to progestin-only or non-hormonal methods and were included in a Cochrane meta-analysis [21]:

1. Medroxyprogesterone acetate (DMPA) 25 mg plus estradiol-cypionate (E2C) 5 mg (Cyclofem®).
2. Dihydroxyprogesterone acetophenide 150g/75 mg plus estradiol enanthate 10/5 mg (Deladroxate).
3. Norethisterone enanthate (NET-EN) 50 mg plus estradiol valerate (E2V) 5 mg (Mesigyna®).

This review found no differences between methods in terms of contraceptive effectiveness, although the studies were all underpowered to detect a difference. Cyclofem® resulted in less amenorrhea and discontinuation due to amenorrhea or all bleeding problems than the injectable containing only DMPA. However, women in the combination-injectable group had higher overall discontinuation rates due to other medical (e.g., headache or not feeling well) or personal reasons.

The Injectable No. 1 that contains hydroxyprogesterone caproate plus E2V is used in China. As a monthly injectable, its failure rate was found to be unacceptably high compared with Mesigyna and Cyclofem [22]. A revised schedule for injection was devised which involved two injections in the first month followed by subsequent injections given 10–12 days after initiation of cyclic bleeding or 28 days from the first injection in the absence of bleeding. With this schedule, the failure rate at 1 year decreased but remained statistically significantly higher for the Injectable No. 1 than Cyclofem (0.77 % vs. 0 %, respectively). Discontinuation rates for bleeding abnormalities were 4.88 %, 8.38 %, and 12.64 % for Mesigyna, Cyclofem, and Injectable No. 1, respectively ($p < 0.001$), which are lower than for progestin-only injectables.

There is very little research on CIC use in adolescents. One prospective observational study evaluated the bleeding patterns of 73 adolescents from 14 to 19 years of age receiving a monthly injectable contraceptive containing norethisterone enanthate 50 mg plus estradiol valerate 5 mg [23]. The continuation rate at 1 year was 52 %, but only one of the 38 teenagers was known to have discontinued the method due to bleeding. Over 70 % of participants found the bleeding pattern to be acceptable at each of four assessment points over the year.

It can be surmised that CICs can provide adolescents with many advantages as it is an effective, discreet method. It is not reliant on daily adherence and is associated with regular menstrual cycles, a rapid washout period after cessation, and a faster return of fertility compared to DMPA. Finally, the subcutaneous CIC that can be self-administered may prove to increase acceptability and compliance among adolescents.

Combined Contraceptive Vaginal Ring
Research into vaginal delivery systems for hormonal contraception began over 40 years ago with a ring that released medroxyprogesterone acetate [24]. Despite decades of development, only two contraceptive vaginal rings (CVRs) have been brought to market: NuvaRing®, a monthly CVR containing etonogestrel and ethinylestradiol, and a progesterone-only vaginal ring marketed under the trade name Progering® [25]. Progering® will be discussed in the section "Progestin-Only Contraception".

A 1 year CVR that contains the non-orally active 19-norprogesterone derivative, Nestorone® (NES), and ethinyl estradiol (EE) has been developed by the Population Council [26]. The device measures 58 mm in overall diameter and 8.4 mm in cross-sectional diameter and is designed for use over 13 cycles (3 weeks in/1 week out). In addition to the convenience of yearly use, the ring does not require refrigeration.

In a multicenter trial involving 150 women, three daily dose combinations of NES/EE were compared in a prototype ring (150 NES/15 EE, 150 NES/20 EE, 200 NES/15 EE) [27]. The pregnancy rates at 1 year were 0 %, 0 %, and 4.7 %, respectively. Bleeding patterns at all doses were excellent, with only 2.4 % of women discontinuing for this reason. Following this trial, the device releasing 150 μg NES and 15 μg EE a day was selected for phase III study. The results of this trial are currently being analyzed (R. Sitruk-Ware, personal communication).

PROGESTIN-ONLY CONTRACEPTION
Implants
Nexplanon® and Jadelle® have been approved by the Food and Drug Administration, but only Nexplanon® is currently marketed in the United States [28]. Jadelle® consists of two rods of levonorgestrel (75 mg in each rod), is licensed for 5 years use, and is similar in price to Nexplanon® [29]. However, the Sino-implant (II) is approximately 60 % less expensive than either Jadelle® or Nexplanon® so deserves particular attention [29].

The Sino-implant (II) has been available for many years in China and Indonesia and is now registered in 15 countries (Ghana, Mozambique, Mongolia, Burkina Faso, China, Indonesia, Fiji, Kenya, Madagascar, Malawi, Mali, Pakistan, Sierra Leone, Uganda, and Zambia). It is currently under review in nine additional countries. The device consists of two rods of levonorgestrel, comparable to Jadelle®, thus sharing the same mechanism of action, but differs in that it is only licensed for 4 years of use [30]. The Sino-implant (II) has first-year probabilities of pregnancy ranging from 0.0 to 0.1 % in randomized controlled trials and cumulative probabilities of 0.9 and 1.06 % in the two trials that presented data for 4 years of use [31]. It was noted that in one study the cumulative probability of pregnancy more than doubled during the fifth year (from 0.9 to 2.1 %), and the authors surmised that this may be why the implant is only approved for 4 years of use in China. The device was also demonstrated to have discontinuation rates due to bleeding similar to other implants [31].

The significantly lower cost of the Sino-implant (II) has the potential to facilitate greater availability in countries where rationing is necessary or where women are required to pay a high up-front fee for private supply, like the United States.

Norethisterone Enanthate (NET-EN) Injectable Contraceptive

The NET-EN injection, Noristerat®, is not available in the United States but is common in the United Kingdom, Europe, Africa, and Central America [32]. Noristerat® is a thick, oily fluid that is drawn up into a syringe, the ampoule should be immersed in warm water before use to reduce the viscosity, and it is administered into the gluteus or deltoid muscle. A single injection lasts for 8 weeks, and according to manufacturer's labeling, it may be repeated once. Noristerat® is, therefore, only recommended as a short-term bridging method, for example, by couples awaiting confirmation of successful sterilization after vasectomy or following teratogenic exposure such as immunization for rubella [33]. However, it is often used for longer periods of time "off label".

A Cochrane review of two randomized controlled trials comparing DMPA with NET-EN concluded that there were no differences in terms of effectiveness, reversibility, and discontinuation patterns, except that women on DMPA were 20 % more likely to develop amenorrhea [34].

Some providers may be concerned about the use of NET-EN in adolescents in view of data demonstrating short-term decreases in BMD (bone mineral density) with DMPA (see Chap. 4). A longitudinal study assessed the differences in BMD over 5 years in women aged 15–19 who were using hormonal contraceptives (combined pill, DMPA, and NET-EN) or who were nonusers [35]. Bone mineral density increased in all groups; however, there were lower BMD increases per annum in NET-EN ($p = 0.050$) and COC users ($p = 0.010$) compared to nonusers. There was no difference between DMPA and nonusers ($p = 0.76$). Recovery of BMD was, however, seen in NET-EN users.

Overall it is unclear whether NET-EN offers any advantages over DMPA for adolescents. It is 20 % less costly compared to DMPA, but its limited duration of use requires 50 % more contacts with healthcare professionals. It may be used as a second option when DMPA is not well tolerated, but this indication is not evidence based.

Desogestrel-Containing Oral Contraceptive Pill (Cerazette®)

Cerazette® received its UK license in 2002. Each tablet contains 75 µg of desogestrel, which is metabolized to etonogestrel [36]. Etonogestrel is a selective progestin with high affinity for progesterone receptors and low affinity for androgen receptors compared to other progestins [37]. A high dose can therefore be used to inhibit ovulation without increasing androgenic side effects. A randomized double-blind trial performed over 13 cycles showed that 75 µg of desogestrel daily was sufficient to inhibit ovulation in 97 % of cycles [38]. This difference is key compared to conventional progestin-only pills (POPs) whose primary mechanism of action is thickening of the cervical mucus to prevent sperm entry and fertilization. This cycle inhibition also allows for a longer window period of 12 h if a pill is missed [39].

A randomized controlled trial of bleeding patterns for Cerazette compared to a levonorgestrel-only pill did not demonstrate improved effectiveness for the desogestrel-only formulation (rate ratio 0.27; 95 % CI: 0.06–1.190) [40, 41]. Bleeding pattern disturbances in the first 90-day reference period of this 1 year trial, including infrequent, frequent, and prolonged bleeding, were up to twice as likely in the desogestrel group [40]. The proportion of women experiencing amenorrhea or infrequent bleeding increased from period one to four but those with frequent bleeding declined with time, eventually becoming less in the levonorgestrel group [40].

Nevertheless, the 12-h window period plus the potential for increased effectiveness with Cerazette has put POPs back on the map as a feasible option for adolescents, especially those who are medically excluded from taking estrogens or intolerant of side effects. An observational study recruited 403 women with estrogen-related side effects during previous combined oral contraception use and made assessments at baseline and 3–4 months after taking Cerazette® [42]. The four estrogen-related symptoms resolved or improved in over 70 % of women; adverse events were low (7–8 %) and satisfaction was very high (90 %).

The Progesterone-Only Vaginal Ring

While not necessarily a leading method for adolescents, the progesterone vaginal ring (PVR) was developed to extend the contraceptive effectiveness of the lactational amenorrhea method. The device is a soft, flexible, doughnut-shaped ring composed of silicone elastomers and micronized progesterone [43]. It has an overall diameter of 58 mm and a cross-sectional diameter of 8.4 mm. The PVR is used continuously over a 3-month period (±2 weeks) and releases an average of 10 g of progesterone a day. The PVR can be taken out for intercourse and cleaning, but must be replaced within 2 h of removal.

Comparative studies have demonstrated the PVR and copper T 380A to have similar effectiveness. The 1 year pregnancy rate in 802 women using the PVR was 1.5 per 100 as compared to 0.5 per 100 among 734 women using the copper T 380A (p = NS) [44]. Overall in clinical trials with the PVR, only 3 of 1,466 breast-feeding women became pregnant while using the device during 10,829 women-months of exposure [43].

In addition to being highly effective, the PVR is very safe with no adverse effects on breast-feeding frequency, milk volume, or infant weight [43]. It also extends the period of lactational amenorrhea, a characteristic appreciated by users and which may be of benefit to women who are anemic after delivery. The proportion of amenorrheic women at 6 months while using the PVR ranges from 67.4–87.4 % compared to 7.4–43.7 % of those using the copper T 380A [44, 45]. Additional advantages of the PVR are comfort, ease of use, and user control [44]. Because the device is designed for use while breast-feeding, weaning is the most common reason for discontinuation (14.7 % at 6 months and 50.8 % at 1 year) [43]. Other reasons for discontinuation by 1 year were frequent device expulsions (8.1 %), finding the ring unpleasant to use (6.9 %), menstrual disturbances (5.8 %), and not having a ring available when replacement was due (1.9 %) [44].

The PVR is currently available in Chile, Peru, Bolivia, Ecuador, Guatemala, and the Dominican Republic [46]. However, the Indian Council of Medical Research and the Population Council are working together to explore the potential for expansion into India [47].

Nestorone®-only vaginal rings were shown to be effective at suppressing ovulation, but high rates of menstrual disturbances precluded further investigation [45]. Another 19-typo: progesterone derivative, ulipristal acetate (UPA, previously known as CDB-2914 or VA-2914), is currently being investigated for use in a non-estrogen-containing CVR. A single oral 30 mg dose of UPA is as effective and potentially more effective than levonorgestrel as an emergency contraceptive [48]. When administered in daily low doses, UPA successfully inhibits ovulation and induces amenorrhea in most women [49]. Two dose-finding studies of CVRs releasing 400–500 and 600–800 µg UPA have been completed [50]. The higher-dose device more successfully suppressed ovulation in 68 % of treatment cycles. Bleeding patterns with this device were very good, however, with the mean number of bleeding or bleeding and spotting days over the 12-week period only 4.16 and 7.51, respectively. Further research is needed to determine the optimal dose of UPA in a CVR formulation.

BARRIER METHODS
Female Condom
The US Food and Drug Administration approved the first female condom (FC1) in 1993 [51]. A redesigned version, the FC2, was launched in 2005 and remains the only female condom available in the United States. The female condom is underused; in the United States less than 2 % of reproductive-aged women have ever used the female condom [52]. Female condoms have a higher cost than male condoms and some women and couples find them difficult or awkward to use. Since 2000, however, new designs of female condoms aimed at increasing acceptability while lowering cost have become available in other countries or are in development [53].

The Cupid female condom (Cupid Ltd, Mumbai, India) is a scented, latex device with an octagonal outer ring and an inner sponge to aid insertion and stabilization [54]. It is the second most commonly marketed female condom after the FC2 (PATH, personal communication). Another female condom developed in India by Medtech Products (Chennai, India) is the VA w.o.w. (worn of woman) also known as V'Amour, L'Amour, or "Reddy female condom" after its designer [54, 55]. Introduced in 2002, it is made of latex and has a soft polyurethane sponge at the end of the pouch, and a firm, flexible triangular outer ring at the open end of the pouch holds the condom against the labia [54]. Notably it has a length of only 90 mm (compared to 170 mm with the FC2) apparently making it perform less well than other female condoms [55]. At present, this device is not being manufactured; negotiations are ongoing to sell patents and potentially renew manufacturing (personal communication, PATH). Although both have CE approval allowing distribution in Europe and are available in several countries, neither has been approved by the WHO PreQualification System and thus is not recommended for public sector procurement by donors [55].

Other devices include the Phoenurse female condom (Condom Bao Medical Polyurethane Corp, Tianjin, China) which is only available in China [55]. The device is made of polyurethane and has an inner and outer ring like the FC1 but is somewhat longer at 180 mm. One study comparing it to the FC1 found similar functionality and acceptability [56]. The Natural Sensations Panty Condom (Natural Sensation Compania Ltd., Bogota, Colombia) is a woman's thong panty with a replaceable panty liner containing a condom made of a synthetic resin [54]. The condom is inserted by the man's penis, and the panty can be reused with new condoms. The Natural Sensations Panty Condom is available in several countries in Central and South America.

One of the most promising new devices is the Woman's Condom developed by the Program for Appropriate Technology in Health (PATH, Seattle, WA, USA) with significant input from potential users. The Woman's Condom is a single-size non-lubricated polyurethane sheath that is 227 mm long and tucked into a capsule which dissolves after insertion [55]. The dissolving capsule is made of polyvinyl alcohol, the same spermicidal material used to make the vaginal contraceptive film. Four foam dots on the body of the condom cling lightly to the vaginal wall ensuring stability. A comparative crossover study of the Woman's Condom and the FC1 found that there was less slippage and breakage with the Woman's Condom and it was more favored by users [57]. A randomized crossover trial in South Africa also found that the Woman's Condom was preferred over the FC2 and V'Amour, though functionality was similar [58]. The Woman's Condom received CE marking in Europe in 2010 and Shanghai FDA approval in 2011 [55]. It is currently in phase III testing in the United States [59].

Cervical Barriers

Condoms remain the gold standard for preventing sexually transmitted infection (STI). However, it is acknowledged that vulnerable and young women may have difficulty negotiating their partner's use of either a male or female condom [60]. Epidemiological and biological evidence suggest that susceptibility to STIs, including HIV, is not evenly distributed throughout the female genital tract but that the cervix is a site of particularly high vulnerability especially in adolescents [61]. Cervical barrier devices may therefore provide some protection against HIV and STIs, especially when used in combination with vaginal microbicides.

The SILCS (PATH, Seattle, WA, USA) is a reusable, dome-shaped silicone diaphragm [62]. It has an anatomically shaped, contoured design for easy placement and removal. It does not require fitting and is described as "one size fits most." It is not yet FDA approved, but a phase II/III contraceptive effectiveness trial has been completed and is under analysis. The acceptability of the SILCS diaphragm was assessed alongside the Ortho All-Flex® diaphragm and FemCap™ in 45 sexually experienced young women (aged 16–21), none of whom had used a diaphragm previously [60]. The participants were randomized to one of the devices, educated on how to use it, and then interviewed about their experiences and preferences. Overall 93 % of participants liked the device they tried, 73 % thought insertion was easy, and 84 % found removal easy. Only 13 % ($n = 6$) said that it was awkward to touch their genital area to insert the device. When asked which device they would like to try in the future, over 50 % in all groups stated they would like to try the SILCS. Sixty-seven percent of participants said their main (hypothetical) reason for using cervical barrier would be that it would prevent both pregnancy and disease.

Very few young women in the United States use female-initiated barrier methods such as female condoms, diaphragms, or cervical caps [63]. This study demonstrates the potential for diaphragm-naive young women to successfully use and find an acceptable cervical barrier and the feasibility of larger studies in those who may benefit from a discreet, woman-controlled dual-protection method.

CONCLUSION

Broadening the range of contraceptive choices for women in order to match their specific requirements is at the core of achieving compliance and preventing unplanned pregnancies and continues to be the key driver behind advances in the contraceptive manufacturing. The methods described in this chapter are already available or could be available in the future thereby increasing options for young women.

REFERENCES

1. Hasson HM. Uterine geometry and IUC performance. In: Hafez ESE, van Os WAA, editors. Medicated intrauterine devices: physiological and clinical aspects. Boston: Martinus Nijhoff Publishers; 1980. p. 11–21.
2. Hasson HM. Clinical studies of the Wing Sound II metrology device. In: Zatuchni GI, Goldsmith A, Sciarra JJ, editors. Intrauterine contraception: advances and future prospects. Philadelphia: Harper & Row; 1984. p. 126–41.
3. Kurz KH. Cavimeter uterine measurements and IUD clinical correlation. In: Zatuchni GI, Goldsmith A, Sciarra JJ, editors.

Intrauterine contraception: advances and future prospects. Philadelphia: Harper & Row; 1984. p. 142–62.

4. Hubacher D. Copper intrauterine device use by nulliparous women: review of side effects. Contraception. 2007;75:S8–11.

5. Farmer M, Webb A. Intrauterine device insertion-related complications: can they be predicted? J Fam Plann Reprod Health Care. 2003;29:227–31.

6. Wildemeersch D. New frameless and framed intrauterine devices and systems—an overview. Contraception. 2007;75:82–92.

7. Otero-Flores JB, Guerrero-Carreno FJ, Vazquez-Estrada LA. A comparative randomized study of three different IUDs in nulliparous Mexican women. Contraception. 2003;67:273–6.

8. Sivin I. Problems in the conduct and analysis of a comparative randomized study of three different IUDs in nulliparous Mexican women. Contraception. 2004;69:259–60.

9. O'Brien P, Kulier R, Helmerhorstc F, Usher-Pateld M, D'Arcanguesd C. Copper-containing, framed intrauterine devices for contraception: a systematic review of randomized controlled trials. Contraception. 2008;77:318–27.

10. Faculty of Sexual and Reproductive Healthcare Clinical Guidance. Intrauterine contraception. Clinical Effectiveness Unit; 2007.

11. Kulier R, O'Brien P, Helmerhorst F, Usher-Patel M, D'Arcangues C. Copper containing, framed intra-uterine devices for contraception. Cochrane Database Syst Rev. 2007;(4):CD005347.

12. Meirika O, Rowec P, Peregoudova A, Piaggioa G, Petzoldd M. for the IUD Research Group at the UNDP/UNFPA/WHO/World Bank Special Programme of Research, Development and Research Training in Human Reproduction. The frameless copper IUD (GyneFix) and the TCu380A IUD: results of an 8-year multicenter randomized comparative trial. Contraception. 2009;80:133–41.

13. www.wms.co.uk/Family_Planning/IUCDs/Nova-T_380_IUD_Intra-Uterine_Device. Accessed 7 Apr 2012.

14. Haugan T, Skjeldestad FE, Halvorsen LE, Kahn H. A randomized trial on the clinical performance of Nova T380 and Gyne T380 Slimline copper IUDs. Contraception. 2007;75:171–6.

15. Bilian X. Chinese experience with intrauterine devices. Contraception. 2007;75(6 Suppl):S31–4.

16. Liu X, Yao M, Ma L, et al. The multi-center comparative clinical trial of the second generation of indomethacin VCu and TCu380A. Reprod Contracept. 2002;1:28–36.

17. Fraser I. Non-contraceptive health benefits of intrauterine hormonal systems. Contraception. 2010;82:396–403.

18. Wildermeersch D, Andrade A. Review of clinical experience with the frameless LNG-IUS for contraception and treatment of heavy menstrual bleeding. Gynecol Endocrinol. 2010;26(5):383–9.

19. Wildermeersch D, Janssens D, Andrade A. The Femilis LNG-IUS: contraceptive performance—an interim analysis. Eur J Contracept Reprod Health Care. 2009;14(2):103–10.

20. www.clinicaltrials.gov/ct2/show/NCT00995150?term=medicines+3 60&rank=1. Accessed 7 Apr 2012.
21. Gallo MF, Grimes DA, Lopez LM, Schulz KF, d'Arcangues C. Combination injectable contraceptives for contraception. Cochrane Database Syst Rev. 2008;(4):CD004568.
22. Sang GW, Shao QX, Ge RS, Ge JL, Chen JK, Song S, Fang KJ, He ML, Luo SY, Chen SF, et al. A multicentred phase III comparative clinical trial of Mesigyna, Cyclofem and Injectable No. 1 given monthly by intramuscular injection to Chinese women. I. Contraceptive efficacy and side effects. Contraception. 1995;51: 167–83.
23. de Bortolotti Mello Jacobucci MS, Guazzelli CA, Barbieri M, Araujo FF, Moron AF. Bleeding patterns of adolescents using a combination contraceptive injection for 1 year. Contraception. 2006;73:594–7.
24. Mishell DR, Lumkin ME. Contraceptive effects of varying doses of progestogen in silastic vaginal rings. Fertil Steril. 1970;21:99–103.
25. Brache V, Faundes A. Contraceptive vaginal rings: a review. Contraception. 2010;82:418–27.
26. http://www.popcouncil.org/pdfs/factsheets/RH_ContraceptiveDev. pdf. Accessed 23 Apr 2012.
27. Sivin I, Mishell Jr DR, Alvarez F, Brache V, Elomaa K, Lähteenmäki P, Massai R, Miranda P, Croxatto H, Dean C, Small M, Nash H, Jackanicz TM. Contraceptive vaginal rings releasing Nestorone and ethinylestradiol: a 1-year dose-finding trial. Contraception. 2005;71:122–9.
28. www.popcouncil.org/what/jadelle.asp. Accessed 10 Apr 2012.
29. Tumlinsona K, Steinerb M, Rademacherb K, Olawoc A, Solomon C, Brattb M. The promise of affordable implants: is cost recovery possible in Kenya? Contraception. 2011;83:88–93.
30. Greene E, Stanback J. Old barriers need not apply: opening doors for new contraceptives in the developing world. Contraception. 2012;85:11–4.
31. Steiner AM, Lopez AL, Grimes D, Cheng L, Shelton J, Trussell J, Farley T, Dorflinger L. Sino-implant (II)—a levonorgestrel-releasing two-rod implant: systematic review of the randomized controlled trials. Contraception. 2010;81:197–201.
32. http://contraception.about.com/od/prescriptionoptions/g/ Noristerat.htm. Accessed 10 Apr 2012.
33. www.medicines.org.uk/emc/medicine/1835/SPC. Accessed 10 Apr 2012.
34. Draper B, Morroni C, Hoffman M, Smit J, Beksinska M, Hpagood J, Van der Merwe L. Depot medroxyprogesterone versus norethisterone enanthate for long-acting progestogenic contraception. Cochrane Database Syst Rev. 2006;(3):CD005214.
35. Beksinska M, Kleinschmidt I, Smit J, Farley T. Bone mineral density in a cohort of adolescents during use of norethisterone enanthate, depot-medroxyprogesterone acetate or combined oral

contraceptives and after discontinuation of norethisterone enanthate. Contraception. 2009;79:345–9.

36. Clinical Effectiveness Unit. Faculty of Family Planning and Reproductive Health Care. New Product Review. 2003; desogestrel-only pill (Cerazette).

37. Kloosterboer HJ, Vonk-Noordegraaf CA, Turpijn EW. Selectivity in progesterone and androgen receptor binding of progestogens used in oral contraception. Contraception. 1988;38:325–32.

38. Rice CF, Killick SR, Dieben TOM, Coelingh Bennick HJT. A comparison of the inhibition of ovulation achieved by desogestrel 75microgrammes and levonorgestrel 30 micrograms daily. Hum Reprod. 1999;14:982–5.

39. Summary of product characteristics for cerazette. www.medicines.org.uk/emc/medicine/10098/SPC/. Accessed 14 Apr 2012.

40. A double-blind study comparing the contraceptive efficacy, acceptability and safety of two progestogen-only pills containing desogestrel 75 micrograms/day or levonorgestrel 30 micrograms/day. Collaborative Study Group on the Desogestrel-containing Progestogen-only Pill. Eur J Contracept Reprod Health Care. 1998; 3(4):169–78.

41. Grimes DA, Lopez LM, O'Brien PA, Raymond EG. Progestin-only pills for contraception. Cochrane Database Syst Rev. 2010;(1): CD007541.

42. Ahrendt HJ, Karckt U, Pichl T, Mueller T, Ernst U. The effects of an oestrogen-free, desogestrel-containing oral contraceptive in women with cyclical symptoms: results from two studies on oestrogen-related symptoms and dysmenorrhea. Eur J Contracept Reprod Health Care. 2007;12(4):354–61.

43. Nath A, Sitruk-Ware R. Progesterone vaginal ring for contraceptive use during lactation. Contraception. 2010;82:428–34.

44. Sivin I, Díaz S, Croxatto HB, Miranda P, Shaaban M, Sayed EH, Xiao B, Wu SC, Du M, Alvarez F, Brache V, Basnayake S, McCarthy T, Lacarra M, Mishell Jr DR, Koetsawang S, Stern J, Jackanicz T. Contraceptives for lactating women: a comparative trial of a progesterone-releasing vaginal ring and the copper T 380A IUD. Contraception. 1997;55:225–32.

45. Brache V, Mishell DR, Lahteenmaki P, Alvarez F, Elomaa K, Jackanicz T, Faundes A. Ovarian function during use of vaginal rings delivering three different doses of Nestorone. Contraception. 2001;63:257–61.

46. Caucus on New and Underused Reproductive Health Technologies. Progesterone-only vaginal ring; 2011. http://www.path.org/publications/files/RHSC_povr_br.pdf. Accessed 8 Apr 2012.

47. Population Council. Progesterone Ring for Lactating Women. http://www.popcouncil.org/projects/252_ProgesteroneRing.asp. Accessed 8 Apr 2012.

48. Glasier AF, Cameron ST, Fine PM, Logan SJ, Casale W, Van Horn J, Sogor L, Blithe DL, Scherrer B, Mathe H, Jaspart A, Ulmann A,

Gainer E. Ulipristal acetate versus levonorgestrel for emergency contraception: a randomised non-inferiority trial and meta-analysis. Lancet. 2010;375:555–62.

49. Chabbert-Buffet N, Pintiaux-Kairis A, Bouchard P, VA2914 Study Group. Effects of the progesterone receptor modulator VA2914 in a continuous low dose on the hypothalamic-pituitary-ovarian axis and endometrium in normal women: a prospective, randomized, placebo-controlled trial. J Clin Endocrinol Metab. 2007;92: 3582–9.

50. Brache V, Sitruk-Ware R, Williams A, Blithe D, Croxatto H, Kumar N, Kumar S, Tsong YY, Sivin I, Nath A, Sussman H, Cochon L, Miranda MJ, Reyes V, Faundes A, Mishell Jr D. Effects of a novel estrogen-free, progesterone receptor modulator contraceptive vaginal ring on inhibition of ovulation, bleeding patterns and endometrium in normal women. Contraception. 2011;85(5): 480–8.

51. Gallo MF, Kilbourne-Brook M, Coffey PS. A review of the effectiveness and acceptability of the female condom for dual protection. Sex Health. 2012;9:18–26.

52. Mosher WD, Martinez GM, Chandra A, Abma JC, Willson SJ. Use of contraception and use of family planning services in the United States: 1982–2002. Adv Data. 2004;350:1–36.

53. Beksinska M, Smith J, Joanis C, Usher-Patel M, Potter W. Female condom technology: new products and regulatory issues. Contraception. 2011;83:316–21.

54. Smita J, Neelam J, Rochelle DY, et al. Comparative acceptability study of the Reality female condom and the version 4 of modified Reddy female condom in India. Contraception. 2005;72:366–71.

55. Mauck C, Joshi S, Schwartz J, Callahan M, Walsh T. Reddy female condom: functional performance of a 90-mm shaft length in two clinical studies. Contraception. 2011;83:466–71.

56. Hou LY, Qiu HY, Zhao YZ, Zeng XS, Cheng YM. A crossover comparison of two types of female condom. Int J Gynaecol Obstet. 2010;108:214–8.

57. Schwartz J, Barnhart K, Creinin MD. Comparative crossover study of the PATH Woman's Condom and the FC Female Condom®. Contraception. 2008;78:465–73.

58. Joanis C, Beksinska M, Hart C, Tweedy K, Linda J, Smit J. Three new female condoms: which do South-African women prefer? Contraception. 2011;83:248–54.

59. World Health Organization. Compendium of new and emerging health technologies. www.whqlibdoc.who.int/hq/2011/WHO_HSS_EHT_DIM_11.02_eng.pdf

60. van der Straten A, Sahin-Hodoglugil N, Clouse K, Mtetwa S, Chirenje MZ. Feasibility and potential acceptability of three cervical barriers among vulnerable young women in Zimbabwe. J Fam Plann Reprod Health Care. 2010;36:13–9.

61. Moench TR, Chipato T, Padian NS. Preventing disease by protecting the cervix: the unexplored promise of internal vaginal barrier devices. AIDS. 2001;15:1595–602.
62. http://www.path.org/publications/files/TS_update_silcs.pdf. Accessed 19 Apr 2012.
63. Martinez G, Copen CE, Abma JC. Teenagers in the United States: sexual activity, contraceptive use, and childbearing, 2006–2010 national survey of family growth. Vital Health Stat 23. 2011;31: 1–35.

Chapter 8
Adolescents Who Are Obese

Bliss Kaneshiro and Alison Edelman

OBESITY IN ADOLESCENTS

Once a problem primarily in adults living in industrialized nations, obesity is now a global epidemic that also affects children, adolescents, and the elderly. Paradoxically, obesity can coexist with undernutrition in the developing world, particularly in urban settings due to the types of food available. In the United States, obesity has been a prominent health concern for several decades. In 2010, the Centers for Disease Control (CDC) reported that more than 33 % of US adults were obese with an additional 35 % meeting criteria for overweight [1].

Body mass index (BMI), expressed as weight in kilograms divided by height in meters squared (kg/m^2), is an objective, standard way to categorize individuals by physical stature. BMI is closely correlated with body fat and the health-related consequences of obesity. However, it overestimates body fat in very muscular individuals and underestimates body fat in the elderly who have less muscle mass [2]. In adults, overweight is defined as having a BMI between 25 and 30 kg/m^2 and obesity as having a BMI of 30 kg/m^2 or higher [2, 3]. These BMI cutoff points

B. Kaneshiro, M.D., M.P.H.
Department of Obstetrics and Gynecology, University of Hawaii,
1319 Punahou Street #824, Honolulu, HI 96826, USA
e-mail: blissk@hawaii.edu

A. Edelman, M.D., M.P.H. (✉)
Department of Obstetrics and Gynecology, Oregon Health and Science University, 3181 SW Sam Jackson, UHN 50, Portland, OR 97239, USA
e-mail: edelmana@ohsu.edu

A. Whitaker and M. Gilliam (eds.), *Contraception for Adolescent and Young Adult Women*, DOI 10.1007/978-1-4614-6579-9_8,
© Springer Science + Business Media New York 2014

TABLE 8.1   Definitions for overweight and obese in adults and children.

Definition	Adults (kg/m²)	Age 2–20 years
Underweight	BMI < 18.5	BMI < 5th percentile for age and sex
Normal	BMI 18.5–24.9	BMI 5th to 85th percentile for age and sex
Overweight	BMI 25.0–29.9	BMI 85th to 95th percentile for age and sex
Obesity	BMI ≥ 30	BMI > 95th percentile for age and sex
Obesity—class I	BMI 30.0–34.9	ᵃ
Obesity—class II	BMI 35.0–39.9	
Obesity—class III	BMI ≥ 40	
Severe obesity	ᵃ	BMI > 120 % of the 95th percentile for age and sex

Data from: http://www.cdc.gov/obesity/childhood/basics.html; http://www.cdc.gov/mmwr/preview/mmwrhtml/mm5917a9.htm; Barlow [66]
ᵃTerm(s) not defined for this age group

are based on epidemiologic studies done primarily in Caucasian populations. Increasing evidence suggests that health-related risks associated with BMI may vary across racial groups [4]. For example, Asians are noted to be at risk for developing weight-related morbidity such as diabetes and dyslipidemia at BMIs lower than 30 kg/m² [5, 6].

BMI is a valid calculation above the age of 2 years [7]. However, obesity is not defined in adolescents and children in the same way it is in adults. Unlike adults, children and adolescents are expected to accumulate both height and weight. Thus, normal BMI for children and adolescents incorporate national standards for both age and gender. The CDC defines an adolescent as obese if she has a BMI greater than or equal to the 95th percentile for her age [8]. An adolescent who has a BMI equal to or greater than the 85th percentile for her age but less than the 95th percentile is considered overweight (Table 8.1). Several online calculators can help clinicians calculate BMI for adolescents (http://apps.nccd.cdc.gov/dnpabmi/). As adolescents near adulthood, the 85th percentile nears a BMI of 25 kg/m² and the 95th percentile nears a BMI of 30 kg/m², thus approaching the same definitions as in adulthood.

The most accurate estimates of the prevalence of obesity come from the National Health and Nutrition Examination Survey

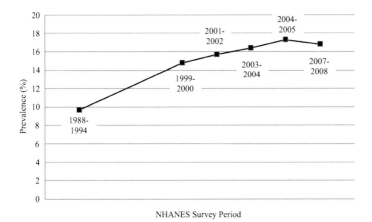

Fig. 8.1 Prevalence of obesity among US females aged 12–19 excluding pregnant adolescents. Data from NHANES Survey. Data from http://www.cdc.gov/nchs/data/hestat/obesity_child_07_08/obesity_child_07_08.htm.

(NHANES) in which height and weight were objectively measured rather than self-reported. In the 1960s and 1970s, it was estimated that 4.6 % of boys and girls age 12–19 years were obese. In the 1980s, rates of obesity in adolescents began to steadily increase. In 2008, it was estimated that the prevalence of obesity in male and female adolescents increased to 18.1 %. Figure 8.1 depicts the prevalence of obesity among females age 12–19 years between 1988 and 2008. Substantial racial differences in BMI exist in adolescents (Fig. 8.2) [9–11]. The prevalence of obesity in adolescent females aged 12–19 was 24.8 % in non-Hispanic black teens, 19.8 % in Hispanic teens, and 14.7 % in non-Hispanic white teens [11].

FACTORS THAT MAY AFFECT THE RISK OF UNINTENDED PREGNANCY IN OBESE AND OVERWEIGHT ADOLESCENTS

The question of whether adolescents with higher body weights are more likely to have an unintended pregnancy has not been studied. However, factors which may affect the risk of unintended pregnancy including the frequency of sexual intercourse have been studied in adolescents. Body weight could affect fecundity as a higher body weight is known to increase the risk of menstrual abnormalities such as polycystic ovarian disease [12, 13]. However, it is important to remember that the majority of obese adolescents will continue to ovulate regularly. Even those who do not ovulate every month are still at risk for unintended pregnancy many times a year.

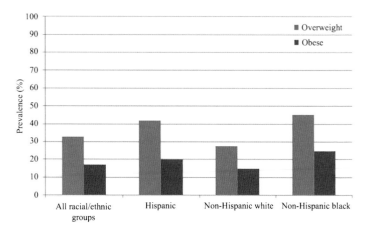

F_{IG}. 8.2   Prevalence of overweight/obese (BMI greater than 85th percentile for age) and obese (BMI greater than 95th percentile for age) among females aged 12–19 years for 2009–2010 (Data from Ogden et al. [11]).

Although data are limited, studies suggest that some differences in sexual behavior between adolescents and young women of differing body weights may exist. A study by Eisenberg et al. found that unmarried women in college who were overweight or obese were more likely to report that their last sexual partner was a stranger, casual acquaintance, or a nonexclusive partner compared to normal weight women (OR 2.70, 95 % CI 1.55, 4.72) [14]. They were also more likely to report being intoxicated during their last-reported act of intercourse (OR 2.25, 95 % CI 1.17, 4.32). However, there was no difference in birth control use (OR 1.20, 95 % CI 0.76, 1.88). Participants in this study also reported on body image satisfaction. Compared to women who were "never" satisfied with their body image, women who were "always" satisfied were not more likely to have a casual partner (OR 1.04, 95 % CI 0.73, 1.50), use birth control (OR1.22, 95 % CI 0.88, 1.70), have multiple same-sex partners (OR 1.14, 95 % CI 0.75, 1.73), or be intoxicated at the time of their last intercourse (OR 0.92, 95 % CI 0.59, 1.43).

A study by Halpern et al. in more than 5,000 white, black, and Hispanic adolescent females found increased frequency of sexual intercourse in adolescent girls of lower body fat indices [15]. In contrast, Akers et al. incorporated the effects of actual BMI and perceived body image on sexual behavior in female adolescents attending high school and found no differences in the likelihood of ever having sex on the basis of BMI [16]. However, girls who perceived themselves as overweight were less likely to have ever had sex. Subjects who had a weight misperceptions (normal weight adolescents who considered themselves overweight) were less likely to report condom use at last intercourse. Among adolescents who were sexually active, those who had weight misperceptions were more likely to have had sex below the age of 13 years.

Compliance with contraception in regards to weight has not been reported in adolescents [17]. Overreporting pill compliance has been documented in many studies and alludes to the propensity of respondents to distort the truth in a way they think will be viewed favorably [18]. A study in adult research participants has introduced the hypothesis of differential pill compliance by body weight [19]. Investigators performed biweekly serum measurement of contraceptive hormone over the course of 4 weeks giving them a reliable way to determine if pills were being ingested. Lack of education, residential poverty, and Hispanic ethnicity were all associated with a higher likelihood of pill noncompliance. When these factors were controlled for, a BMI of 30–39.9 kg/m^2 was also associated with pill noncompliance [adjusted OR 2.8 (1.2–6.9)] [19]. It is essential to note that residential poverty was a strong predictor of pill noncompliance. Thus, it is possible that the results of this study were due to the effect of residual confounding.

OBESITY AND CONTRACEPTIVE EFFICACY IN ADOLESCENTS

The true effect of obesity on inherent drug efficacy is difficult to determine due to the potential confounders discussed previously. Additionally, research in adult women is limited regarding the impact of obesity on contraceptive efficacy, and research on adolescents is nonexistent [20]. For contraceptive methods that rely on the systemic distribution of steroid hormones (pills, patch, ring, injections, implants), a link between obesity and impaired efficacy has not been consistently observed [21–27]. Although population-based studies are somewhat conflicting in their findings, many studies contain only small numbers of obese women and/or a relatively "thin" obese population (a median BMI of 30 mg/kg^2). Additionally, epidemiologic studies are unable to control for drug compliance or fertility status. Better data comes from a recently completed prospective post-marketing study of over 52,000 women and 73,000 women years of oral contraceptive (OC) exposure. This study did demonstrate a slight increased risk of failure (HR 1.5, CI 1.3–1.8) in obese women [23]. Although women below the age of 20 were included in this study, they were not analyzed separately.

Other large epidemiologic studies have reported no increase in risk of contraceptive failure. Analysis of the National Survey of Family Growth and the Oxford-Family Planning Association databases found no association between increased weight and unintended pregnancy in women using progestin-only pills or combined oral contraceptive pills [22, 28, 29]. Another study of women age 18–35, more than half of whom met criteria for being overweight, found no difference in pregnancy rates by BMI when subjects used a low-dose 91-day extended oral contraceptive pill [30]. The crude pregnancy rate for women with a BMI of 25 kg/m^2 or greater was 1.94 % (95 % CI 1.13, 3.08) compared to a rate of 2.22 % (95 % CI 1.34, 3.44) in women with a BMI less than 25 kg/m^2.

Drug efficacy is based on achieving sufficient drug levels to produce a biologic effect. Since obesity affects almost every aspect of drug metabolism, it is plausible this could adversely affect drug levels of steroid hormones and negatively impact contraceptive efficacy [31]. Steroids are absorbed in adipose tissue, potentially resulting in less contraceptive steroid in circulation in individuals with more adipose tissue [32, 33]. Individuals with higher body weights have larger circulating blood volumes which could dilute contraceptive steroid levels [32]. Additionally, higher body weight is associated with an increased metabolic rate including more rapid clearance of hepatically metabolized drugs like hormonal contraceptives [34, 35]. Pharmacokinetic (PK) studies of several hormonal contraceptive methods including oral contraceptives, the etonogestrel implant, and the subcutaneous medroxyprogesterone acetate injection have all demonstrated lower levels of drug in compliant obese users [36–39]. Although it may seem logical to increase hormonal doses for adolescents with a higher body weight, this has not been recommended because this has not been shown to increase efficacy and may impact safety.

The effect of weight on oral contraceptive PK was described in two studies performed in adult women. Edelman et al. measured serum levels of levonorgestrel (LNG) and ethinyl estradiol (EE) following ingestion of low-dose oral contraceptive pills [37]. In obese participants, LNG half-life was significantly altered resulting in a longer period of time required to reach steady state (10 days in obese subjects versus 5 days in subjects with a normal BMI) [37]. A similar study by Westhoff et al. also looked at follicular development, a necessary precursor to ovulation. Compared to women of normal BMI, obese women had lower EE maximum plasma concentrations and area under the concentration curve, a measure of total drug exposure [39]. While lower levels of LNG and higher levels of follicular development were seen in obese women, this was not statistically different from the normal BMI group in this study. A 2012 study did, however, find significant differences in these parameters [40]. The studies had several differences in their methods to account for their slight variation in findings, but both studies suggest that oral contraceptive PK may be altered in obese women. However, it is unclear whether the alterations are large enough to result in decreased contraceptive efficacy [37, 39].

Translation of these PK findings into actual objective evidence of contraceptive failure, i.e., pregnancy, has not been sufficiently studied except in the case of emergency contraception (EC). Both LNG and ulipristal acetate (UPA)-based EC have been shown to be less effective in obese women as compared to women of normal BMI [41]. The risk of failure in UPA-EC users was not statistically significant (OR 2.62, 95 % CI 0.89–7), but for users of LNG-EC, the odds ratio was significantly elevated at OR 4.41, 95 % CI 2.05–9.44. It is interesting to consider that both of these therapies are single-dose treatments, reliant on achieving a certain peak level at a critical time directly prior to ovulation with one dose of the drug.

No data specific to adolescents has been published in regard to the efficacy of the contraceptive patch or ring related to weight or BMI. The contraceptive patch (Ortho Evra, Ortho-McNeil-Janssen Pharmaceuticals, Inc., Raritan, NJ, USA) package label states that the patch may be less effective in women weighing more than 90 kg [42]. This restriction is based on a pooled analysis of three large studies in adult women which found that 30 % of all unintended pregnancies in women using the patch occurred in the 3 % of women who weighed more than 90 kg [43]. Although concerning, these studies were underpowered to determine if an actual risk exists.

The effect of weight on the efficacy of depot medroxyprogesterone acetate (DMPA) via subcutaneous injection has been studied in adult women [36]. Subjects in this 2010 study were recruited into a normal BMI (18.5–24.9 kg/m^2) category, as well as a class I and class II obesity (30.0–39.9 kg/m^2) category and a class III obesity (more than 40.0 kg/m^2) category. Over the course of 26 weeks, DMPA levels tended to be low in classes I and II obese women and were lowest among class III obese women. However, median medroxyprogesterone acetate levels remained above a level needed to prevent ovulation (200 pg/mL) regardless of weight, and there was no evidence of ovulation as determined by progesterone levels.

Literature addressing the efficacy of the etonogestrel implant (Implanon, Organon USA Inc., Roseland, NJ) has been limited to adult women, and most studies have included only women of normal body weight. A PK study of the etonogestrel implant in adult obese women followed for 6 months found circulating levels of hormone lower than that of normal weight historical controls. However, the 2- and 3-year projected serum level remained above the minimum level thought to suppress ovulation. The authors caution that their results cannot be interpreted to conclude that the implant has decreased effectiveness in this population [44]. With the 2-rod LNG-releasing implant (Jadelle, Schering Oy, Turku, Finland), limited studies suggest there may be variability in contraceptive steroid levels by body weight. However, LNG levels appear to be sufficient for effective contraception during the first 5 years of implant use regardless of weight [45]. With the 6-rod LNG implant (Norplant), efficacy was lower in adult women weighing more than 70 kg [46]. However, women in the highest weight category still continued to have an overall high contraceptive efficacy with only 0.86 pregnancies per 100 woman-years estimated over the course of 7 years.

Though not directly studied, BMI should not have an impact on the effectiveness of the copper or hormonal intrauterine device (IUD) for either adults or adolescents as the contraceptive effect is local and not systemic [20]. While placement of an IUD may be more challenging in an overweight or obese, nulliparous adolescent, most placements will not require extraordinary measures. If the insertion is challenging, techniques such as using a large and/ or longer speculum, placing a condom with the tip removed over the speculum for greater vaginal side wall retraction, and/or using ultrasound could be of assistance [20].

Although data continues to emerge regarding obesity's impact on contraceptive efficacy, the bottom line is that the use of contraception in a sexually active woman of any weight or any age will prevent more pregnancies than not using contraception.

SAFETY OF HORMONAL CONTRACEPTIVES IN OVERWEIGHT OR OBESE TEENS

In general, the risks of hormonal contraceptive use are generally exceeded by the risks of pregnancy and the postpartum [47]. The main concern with use of estrogen-containing contraceptives is the risk of venous thromboembolism (VTE). Among children and teens, even in those who have significant risk factors for clotting, the occurrence of VTE is an exceedingly rare event. Even patients with hypercoagulable conditions, such as protein C deficiency, do not typically present with a clot until after the age of 20 years [48]. Data from a longitudinal survey that spanned from 1979 to 2001 reported the baseline rate of VTE in children age 0–17 years to be 0.49 per 10,000 children per year [49]. In teenagers older than 15–17 years of age, the rate in females was 1.49 per 10,000 per year which was higher than the rate found in males (0.81 per 10,000 per year), and this was attributed to teen pregnancy and the postpartum period [49].

The risk of VTE in obese teenagers using combined (estrogen + progestin) hormonal contraceptives is not known but would be hypothesized to be lower than that of adults based on these findings. With low-dose (35 μg EE or less) combined oral contraceptive pills, the risk of VTE in adults is 5–10 cases per 10,000 women per year in nonusers compared to 5–30 cases per 10,000 women per year in users [50]. Obesity is an independent risk factor for VTE with obese adult women having approximately double the baseline risk of VTE compared to women of normal BMI [51]. The risk of VTE in obese, adult women using combined oral contraceptives is yet to be determined. However, because the absolute risk of VTE with estrogen-containing contraceptives is small, the additional risk of obesity is still thought to be much lower than the VTE risk that accompanies pregnancy and the postpartum period [50–53].

No published studies have focused on risks specific to obese women or adolescents who use the contraceptive patch, ring, IUD, or implant. The World Health Organization (WHO) and US Medical Eligibility Criteria (CDC US MEC) for Contraceptive Use utilize an evidence-based classification system to guide clinicians in recommending contraception in women with coexisting medical conditions. Both the WHO and CDC classify the risk of contraceptive use into four categories. All contraceptives are designated either "safe for use with no restrictions" (category 1) or "advantages generally outweigh theoretical or proven risks" (category 2) for obese women from menarche to 18 years without other medical conditions [54, 55] (Table 8.2). Of note, DMPA injection is a category 2 for obese adolescent women because some studies have shown certain teens may be more susceptible to weight gain with the method [47, 56], discussed in more detail below. Further discussion of metabolic effects of hormonal contraception, as well as use in diabetic women, can be found in Chap. 9.

FEARS OF WEIGHT GAIN

Weight gain is commonly cited as a reason for discontinuation and noncompliance with hormonal contraceptives among adolescents [57]. An additional confounder for teens is that they have yet to achieve their adult height and weight and may still be experiencing an increase in both which often get attributed to a contraceptive

TABLE 8.2 US Medical Eligibility Criteria (US MEC) for obesity and bariatric surgery.

	COC	Patch/ ring	POP	DMPA	Implants	LNG-IUD	Cu-IUD
Obesity (BMI ≥ 30 kg/m²)							
Menarche to age <18 years	2	2	1	2	1	1	1
Age > 18 years	2	2	1	1	1	1	1
History of bariatric surgery							
Restrictive procedures	1	1	1	1	1	1	1
Malabsorptive procedures	3	1	3	1	1	1	1

Data from: Medical Eligibility Criteria for Contraceptive Use. http://www. who.int/reproductive-health/publications/mec/ [cited 2012 March 25, 2012] *COC* combined oral contraceptive pill, *POP* progestin-only pills, *DMPA* depot medroxyprogesterone acetate, *LNG-IUD* levonorgestrel IUD, *Cu-IUD* copper IUD [54, 55]

method. In a culture in which young adults commonly turn to the Internet for all types of information, including medical advice, providing evidence-based recommendations to young women when they initiate a contraceptive method can help to decrease misconceptions. The scientific literature indicates that adolescents who use contraceptive pills, patch, ring, implant, or IUD do not experience an increase in body weight or a change in body composition [58, 59].

Studies are conflicting with regard to DMPA causing a weight gain. Many of the studies suffer from poor methodology; specifically, weight is highly individual and therefore weight changes should always be reported as paired data and not as group means—this is a major flaw of most contraception studies reporting weight gain. In regard to adolescents, two retrospective studies found that DMPA use was not associated with increased weight compared to adolescents (aged 12–21 years old) using combined oral contraceptives [60, 61].

Other studies suggest there is a subset of adolescents who are susceptible to weight gain with DMPA use. An observational study compared change in body fat and lean body mass in adolescents aged 12–18 years who were using DMPA to those using no hormonal method [62]. Over 6 months, adolescents using DMPA had a 3.4 % decrease in lean body mass compared to those using a nonhormonal method who had a 0.6 % increase in lean body mass (mean difference –4.0 %, 95 % CI –6.93, –1.07). The DMPA group also had 10.3 % increase in total body fat compared to a decrease in body fat of 0.7 % in adolescents who were using a nonhormonal method (mean difference 11.00 %, 95 % CI 2.64, 19.36). Another observational study noted racial differences in weight gain with black adolescents using DMPA experiencing a higher increase in weight (4.2 % versus 1.2 %) and body fat (12.5 % versus 1.2 %) compared to white adolescents [63]. However, it is unclear whether the weight gain was due to DMPA because this study did not have a control group who was not using DMPA. Teens who gain weight during the first few doses of DMPA use may have a propensity for weight gain with this method. A study by Le et al. reported that adolescents who had a 5 % increase in body weight in the first 6 months of use appeared to gain more weight with DMPA use overall [64].

BARIATRIC SURGERY AND HORMONAL CONTRACEPTION IN TEENS

Although it accounts for less than 1 % of all bariatric procedures [65], bariatric surgery has been described as an option for adolescents with severe obesity (a BMI greater than 120 % of the 95th percentile for age and gender) [66]. A 2005 survey reported that 75 % of bariatric surgeons were planning on performing a bariatric procedure in an adolescent in the upcoming year [67]. The US MEC gives all contraceptives a category 1 rating except for oral contraceptive pills (combined and progestin-only) in women who have had malabsorptive procedures because of a concern for decreased absorption causing lower efficacy (Table 8.2).

CONCLUSION

Few studies have explored contraceptive efficacy and safety in overweight and obese adults and almost none have addressed these issues in adolescents. Given the growing weight demographic in the United States, this is becoming an increasingly important medical concern. However, the lack of research in this area is not a reason to withhold contraceptives to teens. All contraceptives, including hormonal options, appear to be safe in obese and overweight adolescents. Even with some studies suggesting decreased efficacy with oral contraceptive pills as body weight increases, the provision of this form of contraception is certainly better at preventing pregnancies than the use of no contraception. It is important to keep in mind that no matter what the weight, adolescents are at high risk for unplanned pregnancy and have a high unmet need for highly effective contraception. The American College of Obstetricians and Gynecologists (ACOG), WHO, and CDC have identified long-acting reversible methods of contraception like the IUD and the contraceptive implant as "top-tier" contraceptive choices for adolescents [68]. In many instances, use of one of these highly effective contraceptive methods will become the best choice for an adolescent of any weight, whether normal or obese.

REFERENCES

1. Centers for Disease Control. Obesity trends. 2010. Available from: http://www.cdc.gov/obesity/data/trends.html
2. National Institutes of Health (NIH), National Heart, Lung, and Blood Institute's (NHLBI), North American Association for the Study of Obesity (NAASO). The practical guide: identification, evaluation, and treatment of overweight and obesity in adults. Rockville: National Institutes of Health; 2000.
3. Obesity: preventing and managing the global epidemic. Report of a WHO consultation. World Health Organ Tech Rep Ser. 2000;894: i–xii, 1–253.
4. Razak F, Anand SS, Shannon H, Vuksan V, Davis B, Jacobs R, et al. Defining obesity cut points in a multiethnic population. Circulation. 2007;115(16):2111–8.
5. Gray LJ, Yates T, Davies MJ, Brady E, Webb DR, Sattar N, et al. Defining obesity cut-off points for migrant South Asians. PLoS One. 2011;6(10):e26464.
6. WHO Expert Consultation. Appropriate body-mass index for Asian populations and its implications for policy and intervention strategies. Lancet. 2004;363(9403):157–63.
7. Deurenberg P, Weststrate JA, Seidell JC. Body mass index as a measure of body fatness: age- and sex-specific prediction formulas. Br J Nutr. 1991;65(2):105–14.
8. Ogden C, Carroll M. Prevalence of obesity among children and adolescents: United States, trends 1963–1965 through 2007–2008. Center for Disease Control. 2010. Available from: http://www.cdc.gov/nchs/data/hestat/obesity_child_07_08/obesity_child_07_08.htm. Cited 19 Apr 2011.
9. Madsen KA, Weedn AE, Crawford PB. Disparities in peaks, plateaus, and declines in prevalence of high BMI among adolescents. Pediatrics. 2010;126(3):434–42.
10. Haas JS, Lee LB, Kaplan CP, Sonneborn D, Phillips KA, Liang SY. The association of race, socioeconomic status, and health insurance status with the prevalence of overweight among children and adolescents. Am J Public Health. 2003;93(12):2105–10.
11. Ogden CL, Carroll MD, Kit BK, Flegal KM. Prevalence of obesity and trends in body mass index among US children and adolescents, 1999–2010. JAMA. 2012;307(5):483–90.

12. Gordon CM. Menstrual disorders in adolescents. Excess androgens and the polycystic ovary syndrome. Pediatr Clin North Am. 1999; 46(3):519–43.
13. Pelusi C, Pasquali R. Polycystic ovary syndrome in adolescents: pathophysiology and treatment implications. Treat Endocrinol. 2003;2(4):215–30.
14. Eisenberg ME, Neumark-Sztainer D, Lust KD. Weight-related issues and high-risk sexual behaviors among college students. J Am Coll Health. 2005;54(2):95–101.
15. Halpern C, King RB, Oslak SG, Udry JR. Body mass index, dieting, romance, and sexual activity in adolescent girls: relationships over time. J Res Adolesc. 2005;15(4):535–59.
16. Akers AY, Lynch CP, Gold MA, Chang JC, Doswell W, Wiesenfeld HC, et al. Exploring the relationship among weight, race, and sexual behaviors among girls. Pediatrics. 2009;124(5):e913–20.
17. Higginbotham S. Contraceptive considerations in obese women: release date 1 September 2009, SFP Guideline 20091. Contraception. 2009;80(6):583–90.
18. Stuart GS, Grimes DA. Social desirability bias in family planning studies: a neglected problem. Contraception. 2009;80(2):108–12.
19. Westhoff CL, Torgal AT, Mayeda ER, Shimomi N, Stanczyk FZ, Pike MC. Predictors of noncompliance in an oral contraceptive clinical trial. Contraception. 2012;85(5):465–9.
20. Grimes DA, Shields WC. Family planning for obese women: challenges and opportunities. Contraception. 2005;72(1):1–4.
21. Brunner Huber LR, Hogue CJ, Stein AD, Drews C, Zieman M. Body mass index and risk for oral contraceptive failure: a case-cohort study in South Carolina. Ann Epidemiol. 2006;16(8):637–43.
22. Brunner Huber LR, Toth JL. Obesity and oral contraceptive failure: findings from the 2002 National Survey of Family Growth. Am J Epidemiol. 2007;166(11):1306–11.
23. Dinger J, Minh TD, Buttmann N, Bardenheuer K. Effectiveness of oral contraceptive pills in a large U.S. cohort comparing progestogen and regimen. Obstet Gynecol. 2011;117(1):33–40.
24. Dinger JC, Cronin M, Mohner S, Schellschmidt I, Minh TD, Westhoff C. Oral contraceptive effectiveness according to body mass index, weight, age, and other factors. Am J Obstet Gynecol. 2009;201(3):263.e1–9.
25. Holt VL, Cushing-Haugen KL, Daling JR. Body weight and risk of oral contraceptive failure. Obstet Gynecol. 2002;99(5 Pt 1):820–7.
26. Holt VL, Scholes D, Wicklund KG, Cushing-Haugen KL, Daling JR. Body mass index, weight, and oral contraceptive failure risk. Obstet Gynecol. 2005;105(1):46–52.
27. Kaneshiro B, Edelman A, Carlson N, Nichols M, Jensen J. The relationship between body mass index and unintended pregnancy: results from the 2002 National Survey of Family Growth. Contraception. 2008;77(4):234–8.

28. Vessey M. Oral contraceptive failures and body weight: findings in a large cohort study. J Fam Plann Reprod Health Care. 2001;27(2): 90–1.

29. Burkman RT, Fisher AC, Wan GJ, Barnowski CE, LaGuardia KD. Association between efficacy and body weight or body mass index for two low-dose oral contraceptives. Contraception. 2009;79(6): 424–7.

30. Westhoff CL, Hait HI, Reape KZ. Body weight does not impact pregnancy rates during use of a low-dose extended-regimen 91-day oral contraceptive. Contraception. 2012;85(3):235–9.

31. Edelman AB, Cherala G, Stanczyk FZ. Metabolism and pharmacokinetics of contraceptive steroids in obese women: a review. Contraception. 2010;82(4):314–23.

32. Fishman J, Boyar RM, Hellman L. Influence of body weight on estradiol metabolism in young women. J Clin Endocrinol Metab. 1975;41(5):989–91.

33. Stadel BV, Sternthal PM, Schlesselman JJ, Douglas MB, Hall WD, Kaul L, et al. Variation of ethinylestradiol blood levels among healthy women using oral contraceptives. Fertil Steril. 1980;33(3): 257–60.

34. Speerhas R. Drug metabolism in malnutrition and obesity: clinical concerns. Cleve Clin J Med. 1995;62(1):73–5.

35. Ravussin E, Burnand B, Schutz Y, Jequier E. Twenty-four-hour energy expenditure and resting metabolic rate in obese, moderately obese, and control subjects. Am J Clin Nutr. 1982;35(3): 566–73.

36. Segall-Gutierrez P, Taylor D, Liu X, Stanzcyk F, Azen S, Mishell Jr DR. Follicular development and ovulation in extremely obese women receiving depo-medroxyprogesterone acetate subcutaneously. Contraception. 2010;81(6):487–95.

37. Edelman AB, Carlson NE, Cherala G, Munar MY, Stouffer RL, Cameron JL, et al. Impact of obesity on oral contraceptive pharmacokinetics and hypothalamic-pituitary-ovarian activity. Contraception. 2009;80(2):119–27.

38. Gilliam MWS, Chan LN, Mistretta E, Kantor A, Neustadt A. Pharmacokinetics of the etonorgestrel contraceptive implant in obese women (abstract). Contraception. 2011;84(3):305–6.

39. Westhoff CL, Torgal AH, Mayeda ER, Pike MC, Stanczyk FZ. Pharmacokinetics of a combined oral contraceptive in obese and normal-weight women. Contraception. 2010;81(6):474–80.

40. Edelman AB, Cherala G, Murnarb MY, Dubois B, McInnis M, Stanczyk FZ, et al. Prolonged monitoring of ethinyl estradiol and levonorgestrel levels confirms an altered pharmacokinetic profile in obese oral contraceptives users. Contraception. 2013;87(2):220–6. Epub 2012 Nov 12.

41. Glasier A, Cameron ST, Blithe D, Scherrer B, Mathe H, Levy D, et al. Can we identify women at risk of pregnancy despite using emergency contraception? Data from randomized trials of ulipristal acetate and levonorgestrel. Contraception. 2011;84(4):363–7.

42. Ortho Evra Patch Package Label. Available from: http://www. accessdata.fda.gov/drugsatfda_docs/label/2008/021180s026lbl.pdf. Cited 21 Apr 2011.
43. Zieman M, Guillebaud J, Weisberg E, Shangold GA, Fisher AC, Creasy GW. Contraceptive efficacy and cycle control with the Ortho Evra/Evra transdermal system: the analysis of pooled data. Fertil Steril. 2002;77(2 Suppl 2):S13–8.
44. Mornar S, Chan LN, Mistretta S, Neustadt A, Martins S, Gilliam M. Pharmacokinetics of the etonogestrel contraceptive implant in obese women [Comparative Study Research Support, Non-U.S. Gov't Validation Studies]. Am J Obstet Gynecol. 2012;207(2):110. e1–6.
45. Sivin I, Wan L, Ranta S, Alvarez F, Brache V, Mishell Jr DR, et al. Levonorgestrel concentrations during 7 years of continuous use of Jadelle contraceptive implants. Contraception. 2001;64(1):43–9.
46. Sivin I. Contraception with NORPLANT implants. Hum Reprod. 1994;9(10):1818–26.
47. Centers for Disease Control. Medical eligibility criteria for contraceptive use. CDC. 2010. Cited 2 Jan 2012.
48. Lensen RP, Rosendaal FR, Koster T, Allaart CF, de Ronde H, Vandenbroucke JP, et al. Apparent different thrombotic tendency in patients with factor V Leiden and protein C deficiency due to selection of patients. Blood. 1996;88(11):4205–8.
49. Stein PD, Kayali F, Olson RE. Incidence of venous thromboembolism in infants and children: data from the National Hospital Discharge Survey. J Pediatr. 2004;145(4):563–5.
50. Heinemann LA, Dinger JC. Range of published estimates of venous thromboembolism incidence in young women. Contraception. 2007;75(5):328–36.
51. Abdollahi M, Cushman M, Rosendaal FR. Obesity: risk of venous thrombosis and the interaction with coagulation factor levels and oral contraceptive use. Thromb Haemost. 2003;89(3):493–8.
52. Nightingale AL, Lawrenson RA, Simpson EL, Williams TJ, MacRae KD, Farmer RD. The effects of age, body mass index, smoking and general health on the risk of venous thromboembolism in users of combined oral contraceptives. Eur J Contracept Reprod Health Care. 2000;5(4):265–74.
53. Larsen TB, Sorensen HT, Gislum M, Johnsen SP. Maternal smoking, obesity, and risk of venous thromboembolism during pregnancy and the puerperium: a population-based nested case-control study. Thromb Res. 2007;120(4):505–9.
54. Medical Eligibility Criteria for Contraceptive Use. http://www.who.int/reproductive-health/publications/mec/. Cited 25 Mar 2012.
55. Farr S, Folger SG, Paulen M, Tepper N, Whiteman M, Zapata L, et al. U S. medical eligibility criteria for contraceptive use, 2010: adapted from the World Health Organization medical eligibility criteria for contraceptive use, 4th edition. MMWR Recomm Rep. 2010;59:1–86.

56. Bonny AE, Secic M, Cromer B. Early weight gain related to later weight gain in adolescents on depot medroxyprogesterone acetate. Obstet Gynecol. 2011;117(4):793–7.
57. Emans SJ, Grace E, Woods ER, Smith DE, Klein K, Merola J. Adolescents' compliance with the use of oral contraceptives. JAMA. 1987;257(24):3377–81.
58. Reubinoff BE, Grubstein A, Meirow D, Berry E, Schenker JG, Brzezinski A. Effects of low-dose estrogen oral contraceptives on weight, body composition, and fat distribution in young women. Fertil Steril. 1995;63(3):516–21.
59. Lloyd T, Lin HM, Matthews AE, Bentley CM, Legro RS. Oral contraceptive use by teenage women does not affect body composition. Obstet Gynecol. 2002;100(2):235–9.
60. Tuchman LK, Huppert JS, Huang B, Slap GB. Adolescent use of the monthly contraceptive injection. J Pediatr Adolesc Gynecol. 2005;18(4):255–60.
61. Tankeyoon M, Dusitsin N, Poshyachinda V, Larsson-Cohn U. A study of glucose tolerance, serum transaminase and lipids in women using depot-medroxyprogesterone acetate and a combination-type oral contraceptive. Contraception. 1976;14(2):199–214.
62. Bonny AE, Secic M, Cromer BA. A longitudinal comparison of body composition changes in adolescent girls receiving hormonal contraception. J Adolesc Health. 2009;45(4):423–5.
63. Bonny AE, Britto MT, Huang B, Succop P, Slap GB. Weight gain, adiposity, and eating behaviors among adolescent females on depot medroxyprogesterone acetate (DMPA). J Pediatr Adolesc Gynecol. 2004;17(2):109–15.
64. Le YC, Rahman M, Berenson AB. Early weight gain predicting later weight gain among depot medroxyprogesterone acetate users. Obstet Gynecol. 2009;114(2 Pt 1):279–84.
65. Tsai WS, Inge TH, Burd RS. Bariatric surgery in adolescents: recent national trends in use and in-hospital outcome. Arch Pediatr Adolesc Med. 2007;161(3):217–21.
66. Barlow SE. Expert committee recommendations regarding the prevention, assessment, and treatment of child and adolescent overweight and obesity: summary report. Pediatrics. 2007;120 Suppl 4:S164–92.
67. Allen SR, Lawson L, Garcia V, Inge TH. Attitudes of bariatric surgeons concerning adolescent bariatric surgery (ABS). Obes Surg. 2005;15(8):1192–5.
68. American College of Obstetricians and Gynecologists. ACOG Committee Opinion No. 392, December 2007. Intrauterine device and adolescents. Obstet Gynecol. 2007;110(6):1493–5.

Chapter 9
Adolescents with Medical Illness

Elizabeth Janiak and Deborah Bartz

INTRODUCTION

While promoting planned pregnancy is central to the health of all women and their children, ensuring that pregnancies are anticipated and intended is particularly important for those with medical illness. Many chronic diseases heighten the risk for adverse obstetrical and birth outcomes, while pregnancy may also exacerbate disease severity. Young women using certain medications are at risk of resulting congenital anomalies if their regimens are not adjusted before conception. Therefore, it is particularly important to ensure that young women with medical illness have access to contraceptive methods they can use effectively. When working with chronically ill adolescents, it may be helpful to emphasize that the risks of contraception rarely, if ever, outweigh the risks of pregnancy and childbirth.

This chapter covers contraceptive management in illnesses that are either commonly encountered among adolescents and young women, such as migraine headache, or that are of such medical significance that they have great clinical and social impact on a young woman's daily life, such as cystic fibrosis or sickle cell disease. Contraception in the setting of obesity is covered separately in Chap. 8 and for women with disabilities in Chap. 10.

In this chapter, we make frequent reference to the Centers for Disease Control and Prevention's US Medical Eligibility Criteria

E. Janiak, M.A., M.Sc. • D. Bartz, M.D., M.P.H. (✉)
Department of Obstetrics, Gynecology, and Reproductive Biology,
Brigham and Women's Hospital, 75 Francis Street, Boston,
MA 02115, USA
e-mail: ejaniak@partners.org; dbartz@partners.org

A. Whitaker and M. Gilliam (eds.), *Contraception for Adolescent and Young Adult Women*, DOI 10.1007/978-1-4614-6579-9_9,
© Springer Science + Business Media New York 2014

(MEC) for Contraceptive Use, which represent a consensus opinion of experts in family planning and disease management based on the current literature [1]. The US MEC classify contraceptive methods into four categories according to the propriety of their use in particular populations of women and disease settings (Appendix A). The MEC classifications of all common non-barrier contraceptive methods for young women with the illnesses discussed in this chapter are summarized in Appendix B. We do not discuss barrier methods in this chapter. Although there are no medical contraindications to barrier birth control methods, they are associated with high typical-use failure rates. The US MEC states that women with medical conditions associated with a high risk of adverse consequences from unintended pregnancy should be advised that sole use of barrier or behavioral methods may not be an appropriate choice due to high typical-use failure rates [1].

PULMONARY DISEASE
Asthma
Asthma is the most common chronic illness among young people in the United States, with 20 % lifetime and 10 % current prevalence among adolescents [2] versus 7.7 % current prevalence among adults [3]. Black Americans and those living in poverty experience particularly high asthma prevalence among adults, at 11.1 % and 11.6 %, respectively [3]. An estimated 7 % of pregnant women suffer from asthma [4], and while well-controlled asthma has not generally been associated with major adverse maternal and infant health outcomes, prior studies may be biased to underestimate risk due to artificially high medication adherence among study participants [5]. Poorly controlled asthma has been associated with gestational hypertension and preterm birth [6]. Asthmatic patients should, like all patients, be counseled regarding optimal preconception health and medication use during pregnancy according to current best practice guidelines [5].

Recommended Contraceptive Methods and Cautions
for Young Women with Asthma
Women with asthma are generally eligible for any method of contraception, and asthma is not a medical condition included in the US MEC. However, methods that decrease the frequency of menses may be of benefit to these patients. The prevalence of premenstrual asthma, a condition characterized by worsening respiratory symptoms and/or decreased peak flow in the premenstrual period,

has varied between studies from 8.2 to 40 % [7]. Although not proven to reduce premenstrual asthma, practitioners may consider prescribing depot medroxyprogesterone acetate (DMPA), the subdermal implant, or continuous or extended-cycle combined hormonal contraception (CHC) for asthmatic patients with a history of premenstrual asthma in an effort to minimize cyclic hormonal drops that may precipitate asthma aggravation.

Cystic Fibrosis

Approximately 900–1,200 children, or 1 in 2,500 live births, are diagnosed with cystic fibrosis (CF) annually [8]. Due to the increased longevity of patients with CF over the past 50 years, many patients are now living to reproductive age, may require contraception, and may desire pregnancy [9]. Small-scale studies have consistently found that many women with CF use contraception, though they may be less likely to do so than their peers due to misperceptions about fertility and gaps in care [10, 11].

Recommended Contraceptive Methods and Cautions
for Young Women with Cystic Fibrosis

Since CF is a multisystem disease with a spectrum of clinical severity, contraceptive recommendations should be individualized to each patient. The disease effects on the primary organ systems affected in CF (respiratory, gastrointestinal, and genitourinary systems) do not pose any direct contraindication to any contraceptive methods. However, there are several aspects of the disease that should be taken into account during contraceptive counseling. For example, because estrogen can affect endothelial regulators and thrombosis, young women with CF complicated by pulmonary hypertension should avoid CHC [12]. CF patients with severe malabsorption may be steered away from oral contraception due to both a concern of poor steroid absorption and the potential for increased nausea with these medications. Lastly, since bone health may already be compromised by the malabsorption and chronic disease burden of CF, DMPA should be used with caution in this population. Pregnancies in women with CF have been reported in the literature. While the outcomes for the baby are generally good and some mothers do well, others find that CF either complicates the pregnancy or is adversely affected by the pregnancy [13]. Taking all of the above considerations into account, most women with CF should be directed toward highly effective methods of birth control such as long-acting reversible contraception (LARC).

CARDIAC CONDITIONS
Cardiac Anomalies

Though structural defects can develop as a result of infection or myocardial infarction, affected adolescents and young women generally have cardiac anomalies present at birth. The incidence of congenital cardiac anomalies in the United States is low overall, ranging from 0.72 to 4.71 per 10,000 births depending on type [14]. All women with cardiac anomalies should plan and manage pregnancies with caution. The cardiac function of patients with cardiac disease or heart failure is most commonly classified according to the New York Heart Association's functional classes [15]. A woman whose illness is classified as functional class III (comfort at rest but marked limitation of physical activity) or IV (symptomatic at rest and/or inability to carry on any physical activity comfortably) and those with a history of heart failure, transient ischemic attack, or stroke, or with current cyanosis are at particularly heightened risk of adverse neonatal or peripartum outcomes should they become pregnant [16, 17]. However, many patients with cardiac anomalies have healthy pregnancies with planning and monitoring.

Recommended Contraceptive Methods and Cautions
for Young Women with Cardiac Anomalies

The World Health Organization categorizes pregnancy as absolutely contraindicated for women with the following conditions: pulmonary arterial hypertension, severe systemic ventricular dysfunction, previous peripartum cardiomyopathy with any residual impairment of left ventricular function, severe left heart obstruction, and Marfan syndrome with aorta dilated >40 mm [17]. These women should consult with their cardiologist, maternal fetal medicine specialist, and family planning specialist regarding highly effective or permanent contraception, such as the copper and hormonal IUDs, the subdermal implant, or sterilization.

Women with uncomplicated valvular heart disease are eligible for any hormonal or nonhormonal contraceptive method [1]. Women with valvular heart disease complicated by pulmonary hypertension, risk for atrial fibrillation, or a history of subacute bacterial endocarditis should not use estrogen-containing hormonal contraception [1]. All other methods are acceptable for this population. It should be noted that patients at high risk for infective endocarditis who are recommended to use prophylactic antibiotics for dental procedures do not require such prophylaxis for minor gynecologic procedures, such as an IUD insertion [18, 19].

Hypertension

Adolescents and young women can develop secondary hypertension in the setting of obesity, substance abuse, and Turner's syndrome, among other illnesses. Since hypertension increases the risk of myocardial infarction and stroke, the increased risk for these events associated with combined hormonal contraceptive use should be considered during contraceptive counseling. Counseling may need to be multidisciplinary as a means of primary risk reduction of the inciting disease causing the hypertension (such as weight loss in the setting of obesity or recovery in the setting of substance abuse) or in reduction of other concurrent cardiovascular risk factors (such as cessation of smoking).

Recommended Contraceptive Methods and Cautions
for Young Women with Hypertension
If a young woman's hypertension is adequately controlled, combined hormonal methods may be prescribed with careful monitoring when other methods are unacceptable, but other methods are preferred (US MEC Category 3). Women with severe uncontrolled hypertension (systolic ≥ 160 mmHg *or* diastolic ≥ 100 mmHg) or who have hypertension with vascular disease should avoid combined hormonal methods (Category 4). Progestin-only pills (POPs), the subdermal implant, and the levonorgestrel intrauterine system (LNG-IUS) may be prescribed both to women with adequately controlled hypertension (US MEC Category 1) and to women with severe uncontrolled hypertension or with coexisting vascular disease (US MEC Category 2). DMPA requires a bit more caution due to its hypo-estrogenic effect and the resulting reduction in high-density lipoprotein (HDL) levels elicited in patients on this medication, which may negatively impact CVD risk [20, 21]. Therefore, DMPA is US MEC Category 2 for patients with controlled hypertension and Category 3 for patients with uncontrolled disease or co-occurring vascular disease.

Hypertensive combined hormonal contraceptive users are at higher risk of adverse cardiovascular events than hypertensive women who do not use oral contraceptives [22]. For women who are normotensive at baseline, studies have shown that combined hormonal contraceptive use is associated with a small but statistically significant increase in blood pressure (on average 4 mmHg increase in systolic pressure), but that blood pressure generally remains within the normal range and that these elevations return to baseline with discontinuation of oral contraceptives. Oral contraceptive use may contribute to the development of overt hypertension, as seen in the Nurses' Health Study, where the risk ratio for developing hypertension was 1.8 for women on oral contraceptives compared to non-oral contraceptive users [23]. Thus, discontinuation of CHC in young women with labile hypertension may improve blood pressure control [24].

NEUROLOGICAL DISEASE
Seizure Disorder
Epilepsy is among the most common serious illnesses in children and adolescents, with an estimated 1.4 % lifetime prevalence among teenagers [25]. Several comorbid conditions associated with seizure disorder, such as depression and poor social competence [25], may contribute to a heightened vulnerability to unintended pregnancy in this population, underscoring the need for carefully managed contraceptive care. Planned pregnancy is of utmost importance for these patients because prenatal exposure to antiepileptic drugs (AEDs), particularly multiple drugs in combination or at high doses, is associated with a significantly increased risk of a range of congenital abnormalities [26], as well as emerging evidence of possible long-term detrimental impact of in utero exposure to some AEDs on child cognition [27].

Recommended Contraceptive Methods and Cautions
for Women with Seizure Disorder
All major methods of contraception are classified as a Category 1 (no restriction of use) for women with seizure disorders, with the caveat that drug interactions be avoided between a patient's specific anticonvulsant regimen and her chosen birth control method [1]. Some AEDs impair the efficacy of CHC and POPs; consultation with the patient's neurologist may be warranted when prescribing to these patients. For a list of AEDs and hormonal contraceptive interactions, see Table 9.1.

A small number of open-label studies have explored the use of contraceptives to reduce seizure frequency or severity either through the direct effects of hormonal therapy or through the effects of these therapies on the menstrual cycle. Catamenial epilepsy is characterized by the clustering of seizure activity around a phase of the menstrual cycle and is thought to be a result of a precipitous drop in endogenous progesterone [28]. Use of POPs has been reported to reduce catamenial seizures in case reports [29]. A reduction in grand mal seizures was observed in women using DMPA in one small study [30]. This possible association merits further research.

TABLE 9.1   Selected anticonvulsant medication interactions with hormonal contraception.[a]

Anticonvulsants that decrease steroid levels and may decrease hormonal contraceptive efficacy		Anticonvulsants without known interaction and appropriate for use with hormonal contraception	
Generic name	Trade name	Generic name	Trade name
Carbamazepine	Tegretol	Ethosuximide	Zarontin
Felbamate	Felbatol	Gabapentin	Neurontin
Oxcarbazepine	Trileptal	Levetiracetam	
Perampanel		Lamotrigine[b]	
Phenobarbital		Tiagabine	
Phenytoin	Dilantin	Zonisamide	
Primidone	Mysoline		
Topiramate	Topamax		
Vigabatrin			

Data from Karceski [95]

[a]As new evidence emerges on drug interactions frequently, reference to the latest literature on known interactions with a specific patient's anticonvulsant therapy is recommended. The abovementioned interactions would be less significant for contraceptives that do not rely on circulating systemic hormones. Therefore, clinical judgment should be used when considering the levonorgestrel IUD

[b]Plasma concentration of lamotrigine is reduced by use of combined hormonal contraception [96]. If taken in combination with nonenzyme-inducing antiepileptic drugs, there is no known interaction between lamotrigine and CHCs

Non-migrainous Headache

Many adolescents and young women experience tension and migraine headaches. Due to the implications of contraceptive methods for women with migraine versus more benign forms of headache described below, appropriate assessment and diagnosis of headache symptoms in patients presenting for contraceptive care are crucial. For diagnostic criteria for migraine headache with and without aura, see Table 9.2.

Recommended Contraceptive Methods and Cautions
for Young Women with Non-migrainous Headache
There are no contraindications to the initiation of any birth control methods in women with a history of non-migrainous

TABLE 9.2   International Headache Society diagnostic criteria for migraine.

Without aura

A history of ≥5 attacks of 4–72 h (untreated or unsuccessfully treated), not attributed to another disorder, and with the following characteristics:

At least 2 of the following:	At least 1 of the following:
• Unilateral location	• Nausea and/or vomiting
• Moderate to severe pain intensity	• Phono- and photophobia
• Pulsating quality	
• Worsened by physical activity	

With aura

A history of ≥5 migraine headaches as described above, not attributed to another disorder, of which ≥2 must also be accompanied by aura that either co-occurs with onset of headache or is followed within 60 min by headache

Aura is characterized by the following

At least one of the following, but no motor weakness:	At least two of the following
• Fully reversible visual symptoms such as flickering lights, bright spots or zigzags, or loss of vision	• Homonymous visual symptoms and/or unilateral visual symptoms
• Fully reversible sensory symptoms such as tingling sensation or numbness	• At least one symptom develops over ≥5 min and/or a series of symptoms occur sequentially over ≥5 min
• Fully reversible dysphasic speech disturbance	• Duration of each symptom is ≥5 and ≤60 min

Adapted from Headache Classification Subcomittee of the International Headache Society. The international classification of headache disorders: 2nd ed. Cephalalgia. 2004;24(suppl):9–160

headache (US MEC Category 1). Some women complain of new onset or increased severity of benign headache disease following initiation of CHC. Though the evidence for a causal relationship is mixed [31], the perceived side effect of headache remains a common reason women discontinue hormonal contraceptives [32]. Though there is no strong evidence for switching between estrogen-containing methods (e.g., between pill formulations) in this situation, switching to a combined oral contraceptive (COC) with a lower estrogen dose or to a progestin-only method could be attempted to improve symptoms. Additionally, young women may consider continuing on the current method to see if headache frequency declines over time, as headache symptoms have been found to resolve in 66 % of patients by the second month of COC use [33]. The development of new or worsening headache after starting hormonal contraception, while not comfortable for the patient, does not increase health risks associated with contraceptive use, and all methods remain a US MEC Category 1 in this setting. Patients who report new or worsening headache should also be screened for more serious conditions possibly indicated by headache, such as hypertension. Additionally, patients presenting with new headache symptoms while using any hormonal method should be evaluated for migraine headache and discontinue use as appropriate (see below).

Some women using cyclic CHC may experience headache due to estrogen withdrawal. Estrogen withdrawal headache is characterized by the onset of headache within the first 5 days of estrogen cessation (e.g., placebo or withdrawal days) starting after daily exogenous estrogen exposure of at least 3 weeks' duration (e.g., after at least one cycle on the pill, patch, or ring) and resolving within 3 days of headache onset [34]. For many young women, these symptoms can be successfully managed by an increase of estradiol in the withdrawal period or by switching to continuous dosing of COCs or the ring [35, 36].

Migrainous Headache
As defined by the International Headache Society (IHS) [34], migraine is characterized by headache symptoms that last 4–72 h if untreated or unsuccessfully treated, accompanied by a minimum of three additional specific characteristics, as detailed in Table 9.2. Migraine disease has a 1-year prevalence of 7.3 % in adolescents ages 12–17 and 20.4 % in women ages 18–29 [37]. The lifetime incidence is 13 % for women 15–19 years and 22 % for those 20–24 [38]. Due to the implications of migraine on a woman's long-term health and her contraceptive options, clinicians should take care to be accurate when making this diagnosis. Most notably, migraine is an independent risk factor for ischemic stroke, particularly in the setting of full-term pregnancy [39–42]. Though the evidence linking migraine without visual aura (previously termed *common migraine*) and increased stroke risk is mixed, the relationship between migraine with aura (previously termed *complex migraine*) and increased stroke risk is more clearly established [41].

Recommended Contraceptive Methods and Cautions
for Young Women with Migraine

Young women with a history of migraine, with or without aura, are eligible for the copper IUD (US MEC Category 1) and for initiation of steroidal methods that do not contain estrogen, such as POPs (US MEC Category 1 without aura, Category 2 with aura), DMPA, implantable contraception, and the hormonal IUD (US MEC Category 2 with and without aura). Continuation of any progestin-only method in the context of new-onset or worsening migraine with aura indicates a greater US MEC risk category for each of these methods, with POPs, DMPA, subdermal implants, and the LNG-IUS being Category 3 in this context.

CHC is also an option for many women with migraine without aura (US MEC Category 2), which comprises 75 % of migraine disease, provided they do not have other risk factors for stroke, such as obesity or smoking. However, in the context of new-onset migraine without aura after initiation of CHC, these methods should likely be discontinued (US MEC Category 3). If a patient has migraine with aura either before or after initiation, CHC use is contraindicated altogether (Category 4).

Given the wide range of methods that do not contain estrogen, many of which have the added convenience of being long-term and highly effective, such as implantable contraception, DMPA, and both hormonal and nonhormonal IUDs, patients with a history of migraine should generally avoid combined hormonal methods. However, for patients for whom these alternative methods are unacceptable, carefully monitored use of combined hormonal methods may be preferential over the risk of stroke associated with pregnancy. Partnering with the patient's neurologist may be beneficial if combined hormonal methods are being considered for a patient with active migraine disease.

GASTROINTESTINAL DISEASE
Inflammatory Bowel Disease

Incidence of inflammatory bowel disease (IBD) peaks in late adolescence and early adulthood. The prevalence of Crohn's disease is estimated at 43 per 100,000 children and adolescents under age 20 and at 201 per 100,000 adults [43]. The prevalence of ulcerative colitis is estimated at 28 and 238 per 100,000 children/adolescents and adults, respectively [43]. Several large cohort studies and meta-analyses have found women with IBD to be at increased risk for preterm delivery, low birth weight, and maternal health complications [44, 45], highlighting the benefits of ensuring these diseases are well managed before and during pregnancy.

Contraceptive Recommendations and Cautions for Young Women with IBD
Carefully consider disease severity and current treatment regimen when recommending contraceptive methods to young women with IBD. There are no restrictions for the use of IUDs or implants for women with IBD (US MEC Category 1). For women with mild disease, the benefits of combined hormonal and progestin-only contraception generally outweigh the risks (US MEC Category 2). Because of the impact of steroids on bone health, patients receiving this treatment to decrease inflammation associated with IBD should be steered away from DMPA. For patients with severe malabsorptive disease, such as those who have severe disease or have had large sections of their bowels resected, absorption of oral methods may be compromised. In addition, OCPs may produce nausea in some patients and should therefore be avoided for patients trying to optimize oral nutritional intake. Lastly, IBD patients who are at increased risk for VTE due to surgery, immobilization, vitamin deficiency, or fluid depletion should avoid estrogen-containing methods including COCs, the patch, and the ring (US MEC Category 3).

Bariatric Surgery
Currently, nearly half a million bariatric surgeries are performed in North America each year, with the vast majority of these procedures performed on women, 27.3 % of whom are adolescents and young adults at the time of procedure [46, 47]. Since it has been noted in population studies that obese women are less likely to use contraception compared to women in other body mass index (BMI) strata [48], bariatric surgery patients may be at particularly high baseline risk for unintended pregnancy. Bariatric surgery may also result in social, behavioral, and physiologic changes that put women at increased risk for unintended pregnancy [49, 50]. However, due to the rapid weight loss associated with bariatric surgery, pregnancy carries increased risks for at least a year following surgery [49]. Moreover, due to the ongoing possibility of micronutrient deficiency, planned pregnancy and early prenatal care are particularly important in optimizing birth outcomes in this population [51].

Contraceptive Recommendations and Cautions for Young Women
with a History of Bariatric Surgery
Women who have undergone malabsorptive procedures, most notably a Roux-en-Y, should avoid OCPs (US MEC Category 3). However, there is no restriction on contraceptive method in patients who undergo a restrictive gastric procedure, such as the

laparoscopic adjustable gastric band (US MEC Category 1). Given the strong desire to avoid unintended pregnancy in these patients, especially for the first year after surgery, highly effective long-acting methods should be considered and can often be placed at the time of the bariatric procedure.

Liver Disease
In adolescents and young women, liver disease is rare and tends to be transient. It may develop secondarily to Epstein–Barr virus or viral hepatitis, of which hepatitis B (HBV) and hepatitis C (HCV) can produce chronic infections. Due to widespread childhood vaccination, HBV is increasingly rare in the United States, and HCV remains most common among injection drug users, though it can rarely be transmitted through other means [52].

Recommended Contraceptive Methods and Cautions for Young
Women with Liver Disease
For patients with current transient or chronic liver disease of any etiology, disease severity is monitored through liver enzyme titers. Women with acutely impaired liver function due to hepatitis flares should be steered away from initiation of CHC (US MEC Category 3 or 4 depending on disease severity), as proper liver function is necessary for metabolization of these drugs; however, continuation of these methods is a US MEC Category 2 for these patients. Partnering with the patient's hepatologist is recommended for ill patients with compromised liver function. In women with stable carrier or chronic hepatitis, hormonal contraception does not appear to increase the rate or severity of cirrhotic fibrosis, nor does it increase the risk of hepatocellular carcinoma [53, 54]. For these patients and those with mild cirrhosis, use of hormonal contraception and the copper and hormonal IUDs is a US MEC Category 1. For patients with severe cirrhosis, use of combined hormonal methods is contraindicated (US MEC Category 4) and use of progestin-only methods is generally not advised (US MEC Category 3). The copper IUD remains a US MEC Category 1 for these patients.

Diabetes
Among older children and adolescents (ages 10–19 years), the annual incidence of diabetes diagnoses is 18.6 and 8.5 per 100,000 for type 1 and type 2 diabetes, respectively [2]. Given the significant adverse outcomes associated with diabetes in pregnancy, an annual family planning visit is recommended for all diabetics by the American Diabetes Association to help ensure conception occurs

in the context of good glycemic control [55]. However, diabetic women are less likely to receive birth control counseling, prescriptions, or services compared to their nondiabetic peers [56]. This represents a significant unmet need.

Though type 1 diabetes remains more prevalent in children and young adults, the overall population rise in diagnoses of type 2 diabetes and the skyrocketing prevalence of adolescent prediabetes raise concern about any metabolic changes that might be caused by steroidal contraceptive use, particularly by combined hormonal methods [57]. There is no strong evidence that these methods affect carbohydrate metabolism in healthy women [33]. However, a recent systematic review highlighted a general paucity of studies on this subject, as well as a tendency to exclude overweight women from study populations [58] A recent randomized controlled trial stratified by obesity status and comparing two COC regimens helps to fill this gap. This trial found no clinically significant differences in the changes produced by COC use in insulin, glucose, total cholesterol, low-density lipoprotein (LDL), HDL, or triglycerides between the obese and non-obese groups [59]. There is insufficient evidence to recommend against using any contraceptive method in women at risk for diabetes at this time.

Recommended Contraceptive Methods and Cautions for Women with Diabetes
Young women with well-controlled diabetes are generally eligible for any contraceptive method [1]. Insulin insufficiency can occur as part of polycystic ovarian syndrome (PCOS), the symptoms of which are often successfully mitigated with CHC therapy. There is some evidence of increased triglycerides and HDL cholesterol among women with PCOS using COCs, but other metabolic risk factors such as fasting glucose and insulin appear unaffected [60].

Providers may exercise some caution in using DMPA in young women with well-controlled diabetes (US MEC Category 2) for two reasons: (1) the possibility of increased insulin resistance during DMPA use [61] and (2) the possibility of clinically significant adverse effects on bone health among those with type 1 diabetes, given this population's heightened underlying baseline risk of low bone mineral density (BMD), which is theorized to occur secondarily to insulinopenia and low IGF-I levels [62].

Women who are diabetic and have nephropathy, retinopathy, or neuropathy are not candidates for combined hormonal contraceptives (US MEC Category 3 or 4, depending on disease severity), due to their underlying increased risk for arterial or venous thrombotic events. For these patients, DMPA is US MEC Category 3, due to the potential for reduced HDL [1].

HEMATOLOGIC DISEASE
Systemic Lupus Erythematosus

Systemic lupus erythematosus (SLE) is estimated to affect 54 out of 100,000 US adults and 100 out of 100,000 US women [63]. Prevalence of SLE is much higher among African-Americans, with estimated rates for African-American women of 406–694 per 100,000 in some US regions [64]. SLE affects multiple organ systems, and practitioners should confer with the rheumatologist or other specialists working with patients with more severe disease or secondary conditions such as end-stage renal disease. Among younger women with quiescent or mild active SLE, the primary concern in selecting contraception is hematologic parameters, particularly the presence in some patients of positive antiphospholipid antibodies.

Recommended Contraceptive Methods and Cautions for Women with SLE

A recent systematic review of the evidence found that women with SLE are generally good candidates for any contraceptive method, with the risks of unintended pregnancy usually far outweighing the risks entailed by using most methods [65]. This is in part because pregnancy is associated with increased disease activity, particularly among women with moderate to severe disease at conception, whereas no link between contraceptive use and increased disease severity has been found (though the latter potential association has primarily been tested only in COC users) [66]. Among women with SLE with positive or unknown antiphospholipid antibodies, the copper IUD is a US MEC Category 1, and levonorgestrel-only methods are a US MEC Category 3. In these patients, use of combined hormonal methods is contraindicated (US MEC Category 4). For all other SLE patients, combined hormonal methods, POPs, the subdermal implant, and LNG-IUS are a US MEC Category 2. For women with SLE and severe thrombocytopenia, DMPA and the Cu-IUD are a Category 3 for initiation and 2 for continuation. Like other patients with menorrhagia, women with SLE and this condition may benefit from use of contraceptive methods that reduce menstrual bleeding.

Sickle Cell Disease

Sickle cell disease affects an estimated 90,000–100,000 Americans, including 1 out of 500 African-Americans [2]. The disease is primarily diagnosed early in life. Childhood mortality associated with sickle cell disease has dramatically decreased in recent decades [67], resulting in a higher proportion of affected patients living to reproductive age and requiring contraception.

Recommendations and Cautions for Young Women with Sickle Cell Disease
Systematic reviews of the literature have consistently reported that CHC, progestin-only contraception, and IUDs have not been associated with adverse events among women with sickle cell disease [68–70]. There is moderate evidence that DMPA use reduces both the number and severity of sickle cell crises [71, 72]. Additionally, one small nonrandomized trial found a decrease in sickle cell crises and in clinical symptoms among subdermal implant users [73]. The evidence on combined hormonal methods' effects on sickle cell crises is inconsistent [71, 74]. Despite the lack of convincing evidence that the ameliorative effect produced by DMPA is also produced by use of OCPs, the patch, ring, or implant, the similarity in formulation and mechanism of action of these drugs suggests sickle cell patients may benefit from any hormonal method. DMPA also has the added benefit of inducing amenorrhea in many patients within the first year of use, which may be beneficial to the hematologic profile of these women who routinely suffer from moderate to severe anemia from their sickle cell disease. Although there is concern for increased risk for blood loss with use of the copper IUD, there is no evidence that this IUD has consistent detrimental effect on hematological parameters, and its use in patients with anemia is not contraindicated (US MEC Category 2).

von Willebrand Disease
Decreased level or impaired functionality of von Willebrand factor is estimated to affect 1 % of the population [75], and many affected women who are identified as having von Willebrand disease (VWD) are diagnosed in adolescence during evaluation for heavy or prolonged menses.

Recommendations and Cautions for Young Women with von Willebrand Disease
Women with VWD are at risk for developing hemorrhagic cysts and may therefore benefit from the methods that most effectively shut down ovulation: the contraceptive implant and DMPA. DMPA has the added benefit of thinning the endometrial lining and decreasing menstrual flow, a benefit of the LNG-IUS as well. Patients considering these methods should be mindful of the possibility of heavier menstrual bleeding for a period of time following method initiation. While no method is explicitly contraindicated for VWD patients, the copper IUD may not be appropriate since it can also produce heavier menses than what the patient may already be experiencing.

Deep Vein Thrombosis Risk Factors
Young women may be at risk for deep vein thrombosis (DVT) from a variety of conditions, including SLE, known thrombogenic mutations, cancer, and prolonged immobilization for any reason. Evaluating the propriety of any given method requires assessing the individual's level of risk.

Recommendations and Cautions for Young Women with DVT Risk Factors
Young women with a history of DVT due to an underlying chronic condition should avoid combined hormonal contraceptives, due to the unacceptable cumulative risk of thrombosis with estrogen use. Women with a history of DVT in the setting of a transient risk that has since been ameliorated (such as a temporary period of immobilization that has ended), and no additional risk factors, may be prescribed with combined methods with careful monitoring if other methods are unacceptable to the patient (US MEC Category 3). Known thrombogenic mutations are an absolute contraindication to combined hormonal contraceptive use (US MEC Category 4), but routine screening is not recommended due to the rarity of these conditions and the high cost of screening. A family history of DVT does not prohibit use of combined methods (US MEC Category 2). Progestin-only and nonhormonal methods may be prescribed to patients with risk factors for DVT as well as with a personal history of DVT with minimal concern (US MEC Category 2 and Category 1, respectively).

MENTAL ILLNESS
Depression
Among US women ages 15–24, past-year prevalence of major depression has been estimated at 16.1 % [76], with a trend toward increasing prevalence in recent age cohorts [77]. Evidences of adverse effects of prenatal maternal depressive symptoms on birth and infant health outcomes are mixed [78]. However, depression is associated with poor prenatal health behaviors and is a risk factor for unintended pregnancy, which is in turn associated with many adverse maternal and child health outcomes [79–81]. Newly pregnant women taking certain antidepressant medications are also at risk of the teratogenic effects of some of these drugs in early fetal development.

Recommended Contraceptive Methods and Cautions for Women with Depression
No method is contraindicated for women with a history or current diagnosis of a depressive disorder, with all major hormonal and nonhormonal methods being classified as a US MEC Category 1 for women with these diseases. However, these classifications are

only generalizable to a straightforward diagnosis of depression; data on the effects of hormonal methods on patients with bipolar disorder or postpartum depression are lacking [1]. A causal relationship between hormonal contraceptive use and mood change has not been established. Some studies demonstrate an association between DMPA use and heightened risk of depressive symptoms [82], while others find no association [83] or a protective effect [84]. Due to the conflicting evidence that DMPA can worsen symptoms of depression in some patients, and particularly because the effects of DMPA are typically felt for months following injection, providers may favor other safer and more easily discontinued methods for this population [85]. Despite the conflicting evidence, perceived side effects, including mood changes, remain the most common reasons for discontinuation of DMPA and OCPs nationally in the United States [31].

Disordered Eating
Disordered eating is among the most common illnesses among female adolescents and young adults, with prevalence of extreme weight control behaviors among young women estimated as high as 20 % [86]. Eating disorders are associated with elevated risk of preterm birth, low birth weight, and cesarean delivery [87].

Recommended Contraceptive Methods and Cautions
for Women with Disordered Eating
Among patients with bulimia there is mixed evidence possibly indicating exacerbation of disease symptoms in the premenstrual period [88]. Therefore, bulimic patients may benefit from disease symptom regulation through the reduction of hormonal fluctuations associated with menses by choosing a contraceptive that prolongs the time between withdrawal periods.

Because many patients with anorexia nervosa (AN) experience amenorrhea and may not use contraception, the side effects of contraceptive methods among this population are generally understudied [88]. Women with AN may benefit from COC use, which has been demonstrated to prevent bone loss in this population in a randomized controlled trial [89]. Clinicians managing AN may also choose COC therapy in conjunction with other therapies such as recombinant human IGF-I in order to augment the effect of the latter drug in reversing BMD loss [90]. For patients with AN, DMPA is not advised due to its adverse impact on BMD. Generally DMPA is safe for young women, including teenagers, with no increased risk for clinically significant outcomes such as fragility fractures and with any bone loss experienced during method use being reversible over the long term [85, 91, 92]. However, because patients with AN are at risk for osteopenia, any temporary decline in BMD associated with DMPA may be clinically significant in this population. Given the lack of RCTs measuring the impact of DMPA on fractures, the risks are unclear and caution is merited [93]. Any patients who present with disordered eating should also be screened for major depression, a comorbidity with 40 % prevalence in this population [94], and managed according to that diagnosis as applicable (see Depression, above).

REFERENCES

1. Centers for Disease Control and Prevention. U.S. medical eligibility criteria for contraceptive use, 2010. MMWR. 2010;59(RR-4):i-85.
2. Centers for Disease Control and Prevention. National diabetes fact sheet: national estimates and general information on diabetes and prediabetes in the United States, 2011. Atlanta, GA: U.S. Department of Health and Human Services, Centers for Disease Control and Prevention; 2011.
3. Akinbami LJ, Moorman JE, Liu X. Asthma prevalence, health care use, and mortality: United States, 2005–2009. National health statistics reports; no 32. Hyattsville, MD: National Center for Health Statistics; 2011.
4. D'Angelo D, Williams L, Morrow B, Cox S, Harris N, Harrison L. Preconception and interconception health status of women who recently gave birth to a live-born infant—Pregnancy Risk Assessment Monitoring System (PRAMS), United States, 26 reporting areas, 2004. MMWR Surveill Summ. 2007;56(10):1–35. Erratum in: MMWR Morb Mortal Wkly Rep. 2008;57(16):436.
5. American College of Obstetricians and Gynecologists. Asthma in pregnancy, ACOG practice bulletin no. 90. Obstet Gynecol. 2008;111(2 Pt 1):457–64.
6. Schatz M, Dombrowski MP, Wise R, Momirova V, Landon M, Mabie W, et al. Spirometry is related to perinatal outcomes in pregnant women with asthma. Am J Obstet Gynecol. 2006;194(1):120–6.
7. Tan KS. Premenstrual asthma: epidemiology, pathogenesis and treatment. Drugs. 2001;61(14):2079–86.
8. Cystic Fibrosis Foundation. Cystic Fibrosis Foundation patient registry 2010 annual data report. Bethesda, MD: Cystic Fibrosis Foundation; 2012.
9. Tsang A, Moriarty C, Towns S. Contraception, communication and counseling for sexuality and reproductive health in adolescents and young adults with CF. Paediatr Respir Rev. 2010;11:84–9.
10. Plant BJ, Goss CH, Tonelli MR, McDonald G, Black RA, Aitken ML. Contraceptive practices in women with cystic fibrosis. J Cyst Fibros. 2008;7(5):412–4.
11. Sawyer SM, Phelan PD, Bowes G. Reproductive health in young women with cystic fibrosis: knowledge, behavior and attitudes. J Adolesc Health. 1995;17(1):46–50.

12. Townsend EA, Miller VM, Prakash YS. Sex differences and sex steroids in lung health and disease. Endocr Rev. 2012;33(1):1–47.
13. Simcox AM, Duff AJ, Morton AM, Edenborough FP, Conway SP, Hewison J. Decision making about reproduction and pregnancy by women with cystic fibrosis. Br J Hosp Med. 2009;70(11):639–43.
14. Parker SE, Mai CT, Canfield MA, Rickard R, Wang Y, Meyer RE, et al. Updated National Birth Prevalence estimates for selected birth defects in the United States, 2004–2006. Birth Defects Res A Clin Mol Teratol. 2010;88(12):1008–16.
15. Criteria Committee of the New York Heart Association. Nomenclature and criteria for diagnosis of diseases of the heart and blood vessels. Boston: Little Brown; 1964.
16. Sui SC, Sermer M, Colman JM, Alvarez AN, Mercier L, Morton BC. Prospective multicenter study of pregnancy outcomes in women with heart disease. Circulation. 2001;104:515–21.
17. Thorne S, MacGregor A, Nelson-Piercy C. Risks of contraception and pregnancy in heart disease. Heart. 2006;92:1520–5.
18. Nishimura RA, Carabello BA, Faxon DP, Freed MD, Lytle BW, O'Gara PT, et al. ACC/AHA 2008 Guideline update on valvular heart disease: focused update on infective endocarditis: a report of the American College of Cardiology/American Heart Association Task Force on Practice Guidelines endorsed by the Society of Cardiovascular Anesthesiologists, Society for Cardiovascular Angiography and Interventions, and Society of Thoracic Surgeons. J Am Coll Cardiol. 2008;52(8):676–85.
19. Wilson W, Taubert KA, Gewitz M, Lockhart PB, Baddour LM, Levison M, et al. Prevention of infective endocarditis: guidelines from the American Heart Association: a guideline from the American Heart Association Rheumatic Fever, Endocarditis, and Kawasaki Disease Committee, Council on Cardiovascular Disease in the Young, and the Council on Clinical Cardiology, Council on Cardiovascular Surgery and Anesthesia, and the Quality of Care and Outcomes Research Interdisciplinary Working Group. Circulation. 2007;116:1736–54.
20. Berenson AB, Rahman M, Wilkinson G. Effect of injectable and oral contraceptives on serum lipids. Obstet Gynecol. 2009;114(4):786–94.
21. Kongsayreepong R, Chutivongse S, George P, Joyce S, McCone JM, Garza-Flores J, et al. A multicentre comparative study of serum lipids and apolipoproteins in long-term users of DMPA and a control group of IUD users. World Health Organization. Task Force on Long-Acting Systemic Agents for Fertility Regulation Special Programme of Research, Development and Research Training in Human Reproduction. Contraception. 1993;47(2):177–91.
22. Curtis KM, Mohllajee AP, Martins SL, Peterson HB. Combined oral contraceptive use among women with hypertension: a systematic review. Contraception. 2006;73(2):179–88.
23. Pollara T, Kelsberg G, Safranek S, Schrager S. Clinical inquiries. What is the risk of adverse outcomes in a woman who develops mild hypertension from OCs? J Fam Pract. 2006;55(11):986–8.

24. Lubianca JN, Moreira LB, Gus M, Fuchs FD. Stopping oral contraceptives: an effective blood pressure-lowering intervention in women with hypertension. J Hum Hypertens. 2005;19:451–5.

25. Russ SA, Larson K, Halfon N. A national profile of childhood epilepsy and seizure disorder. Pediatrics. 2012;129(2):256–64.

26. Adab N, Tudur Smith C, Vinten J, Williamson PR, Winterbottom JB. Common antiepileptic drugs in pregnancy in women with epilepsy. Cochrane Database Syst Rev. 2004;(3):CD004848.

27. Banach R, Boskovic R, Einarson T, Koren G. Long-term developmental outcome of children of women with epilepsy, unexposed or exposed prenatally to antiepileptic drugs: a meta-analysis of cohort studies. Drug Saf. 2010;33(1):73–9.

28. Herzog AG. Catamenial epilepsy: definition, prevalence pathophysiology and treatment. Seizure. 2008;17(2):151–9.

29. Verrotti A, Laus M, Coppola G, Parisi P, Mohn A, Chiarelli F. Catamenial epilepsy: hormonal aspects. Gynecol Endocrinol. 2010;26(11):783–90.

30. Mattson RH, Cramer JA, Caldwell BV, Siconolfi BC. Treatment of seizures with medroxyprogesterone acetate: preliminary report. Neurology. 1984;34(9):1255–8.

31. Loder EW, Buse DC, Golub JR. Headache as a side effect of combination estrogen-progestin oral contraceptives: a systematic review. Am J Obstet Gynecol. 2005;193(3 Pt 1):636–49.

32. Mosher WD, Jones J. Use of contraception in the United States: 1982–2008. Vital Health Stat 23. 2010;(29). Hyattsville, MD: National Center for Health Statistics.

33. Nelson AL, Cwiak C. Combined oral contraceptives. In: Hatcher RA, Trusseull J, Nelson AL, Cates W, Kowal D, Policar MS, editors. Contraceptive technology. New York: Ardent Media, Inc.; 2011. p. 249–341.

34. Headache Classification Subcommittee of the International Headache Society. The international classification of headache disorders: 2nd ed. Cephalalgia. 2004;24 Suppl 1:9–160.

35. Edelman A, Gallo MF, Nichols MD, Jensen JT, Schulz KF, Grimes DA. Continuous versus cyclic use of combined oral contraceptives for contraception: systematic Cochrane review of randomized controlled trials. Hum Reprod. 2006;21(3):573–8.

36. MacGregor EA, Hackshaw A. Prevention of migraine in the pill-free interval of combined oral contraceptives: a double-blind, placebo-controlled pilot study using natural oestrogen supplements. J Fam Plann Reprod Health Care. 2002;28(1):27–31.

37. Lipton RB, Bigal ME, Diamond M, Freitag F, Reed ML, Stewart WF, on behalf of the AMP Advisory Group. Migraine prevalence, disease burden, and the need for preventive therapy. Neurology. 2007;68:343–9.

38. Stewart WF, Wood C, Reed ML, Roy J, Lipton RB, AMPP Advisory Group. Cumulative lifetime migraine incidence in women and men. Cephalalgia. 2008;28(11):1170–8.

39. James AH, Bushnell CD, Jamison MG, Myers ER. Incidence and risk factors for stroke in pregnancy and the puerperium. Obstet Gynecol. 2005;106(3):509–16.
40. Kittner SJ, Stern BJ, Feeser BR, Hebel R, Nagey DA, Buchholz DW, et al. Pregnancy and the risk of stroke. N Engl J Med. 1996;335(11):768.
41. MacGregor EA. Migraine and use of combined hormonal contraceptives: a clinical review. J Fam Plann Reprod Health Care. 2007;33:159–69.
42. Pathan M, Kittner SJ. Pregnancy and stroke. Curr Neurol Neurosci Rep. 2003;3(1):27–31.
43. Kappelman MD, Rifas-Shiman SL, Kleinman K, Ollendorf D, Bousvaros A, Grand RJ, et al. Prevalence and geographic distribution of Crohn's disease and ulcerative colitis in the United States. Clin Gastroenterol Hepatol. 2007;5(12):1424–9.
44. Cornish J, Tan E, Teare J, Teoh TG, Rai R, Clark SK, Tekkis PP. A meta-analysis on the influence of inflammatory bowel disease on pregnancy. Gut. 2007;56(6):830–7.
45. Nguyen GC, Boudreau H, Harris ML, Maxwell CV. Outcomes of obstetric hospitalizations among women with inflammatory bowel disease in the United States. Clin Gastroenterol Hepatol. 2009;7(3):329–34.
46. Buchwald H, Oien DM. Metabolic/bariatric surgery Worldwide 2008. Obes Surg. 2009;19(12):1605–11.
47. Santry HP, Gillen DL, Lauderdale DS. Trends in bariatric surgical procedures. JAMA. 2005;294(15):1909–17.
48. Society of Family Planning. Contraceptive considerations in obese women. Contraception. 2009;80:583–90.
49. American College of Obstetricians and Gynecologists. Bariatric surgery and pregnancy, ACOG practice bulletin no. 105. Obstet Gynecol. 2009;113(6):1405–13.
50. Teitelman M, Grotegut CA, Williams NN, Lewis JD. The impact of bariatric surgery on menstrual patterns. Obes Surg. 2006;16(11):1457–63.
51. Ledoux S, Msika S, Moussa F, Larger E, Boudou P, Salomon L, et al. Comparison of nutritional consequences of conventional therapy of obesity, adjustable gastric banding, and gastric bypass. Obes Surg. 2006;16(8):1041–9.
52. Daniels D, Grytdal S, Wasley A. Surveillance for acute viral hepatitis—United States, 2007. MMWR Surveill Summ. 2009;58(3):1.
53. Di Martino V, Lebray P, Myers RP, Pannier E, Paradis V, Charlotte F, et al. Progression of liver fibrosis in women infected with hepatitis C: long-term benefit of estrogen exposure. Hepatology. 2004;40(6):1426–33.
54. Libbrecht L, Craninx M, Nevens F, Desmet V, Roskams T. Predictive value of liver cell dysplasia for development of hepatocellular carcinoma in patients with non-cirrhotic and cirrhotic chronic viral hepatitis. Histopathology. 2001;39(1):66–73.

55. American Diabetes Association. Position statement. Standards of medical care in diabetes—2012. Diabetes Care. 2012;35 Suppl 1:S11–63.
56. Schwarz EB, Postlethwaite D, Hung YY, Lantzman E, Armstrong MA, Horberg MA. Provision of contraceptive services to women with diabetes mellitus. J Gen Intern Med. 2012;27(2):196–201.
57. May AL, Kuklina EV, Yoon PW. Prevalence of cardiovascular disease risk factors among US adolescents, 1999–2008. Pediatrics. 2012;129:1035–41.
58. Lopez LM, Grimes DA, Chen-Mok M, Westhoff C, Edelman A, Helmerhorst FM. Hormonal contraceptives for contraception in overweight or obese women. Cochrane Database Syst Rev. 2009;(7):CD008452.
59. Beasley A, Estes C, Guerrero J, Westhoff C. The effect of obesity and low-dose oral contraceptives on carbohydrate and lipid metabolism. Contraception. 2012;85(5):446–52.
60. Halperin IJ, Kumar SS, Stroup DF, Laredo SE. The association between the combined oral contraceptive pill and insulin resistance, dysglycemia and dyslipidemia in women with polycystic ovary syndrome: a systematic review and meta-analysis of observational studies. Hum Reprod. 2011;26(1):191–201.
61. Kahn HS, Curtis KM, Marchbanks PA. Effects of injectable or implantable progestin-only contraceptives on insulin-glucose metabolism and diabetes risk. Diabetes Care. 2003;26(1):216–25.
62. Mastrandrea LD, Wactawski-Wende J, Donahue RP, Hovey KM, Clark A, Quattrin T. Young women with type 1 diabetes have lower bone mineral density that persists over time. Diabetes Care. 2008;31(9):1729–35.
63. Ward MM. Prevalence of physician-diagnosed systemic lupus erythematosus in the United States: results from the third national health and nutrition examination survey. J Womens Health. 2004;13(6):713–8.
64. Chakravarty EF, Bush TM, Manzi S, Clarke AE, Ward MM. Prevalence of adult systemic lupus erythematosus in California and Pennsylvania in 2000: estimates obtained using hospitalization data. Arthritis Rheum. 2007;56(6):2092–4.
65. Culwell KR, Curtis KM, del Carmen Cravioto M. Safety of contraceptive method use among women with systemic lupus erythematosus: a systematic review. Obstet Gynecol. 2009;114(2 Pt 1):341–53.
66. Culwell KR, Curtis KM. Contraception for women with systemic lupus erythematosus. J Fam Plann Reprod Health Care. 2013;39:9–11.
67. Yanni E, Grosse SD, Yang QH, Olney RS. Trends in pediatric sickle cell disease-related mortality in the United States, 1983–2002. J Pediatr. 2009;154(4):541–5.
68. Legardy JK, Curtis KM. Progestogen-only contraceptive use among women with sickle cell anemia: a systematic review. Contraception. 2006;73(2):195–204.

69. Manchikanti Gomez A, Grimes DA, Lopez LM, Schulz KF. Steroid hormones for contraception in women with sickle cell disease. Cochrane Database Syst Rev. 2007;(2):CD006261.
70. Haddad LB, Curtis KM, Legardy-Williams JK, Cwiak C, Jamieson DJ. Contraception for individuals with sickle cell disease: a systematic review of the literature. Contraception. 2012;85(6):527–37.
71. de Abood M, de Castillo Z, Guerrero F, Espino M, Austin KL. Effect of Depo-Provera or Microgynon on the painful crises of sickle cell anemia patients. Contraception. 1997;56(5):313–6.
72. De Ceulaer K, Gruber C, Hayes R, Serjeant GR. Medroxyprogesterone acetate and homozygous sickle-cell disease. Lancet. 1982;2:229–31.
73. Nascimento Mde L, Ladipo OA, Coutinho EM. Nomegestrol acetate contraceptive implant use by women with sickle cell disease. Clin Pharmacol Ther. 1998;64(4):433–8.
74. Howard RJ, Lillis C, Tuck SM. Contraceptives, counselling, and pregnancy in women with sickle cell disease. BMJ. 1993;306(6894):1735–7.
75. Sadler JE, Mannucci PM, Berntorp E, Bochkov N, Boulyjenkov V, Ginsburg D, et al. Impact, diagnosis and treatment of von Willebrand disease. Thromb Haemost. 2000;84:160–74.
76. Kessler RC, Walters EE. Epidemiology of DSM-III-R major depression and minor depression among adolescents and young adults in the National Comorbidity Survey. Depress Anxiety. 1998;7(1):3–14.
77. Kessler RC, Berglund P, Demler O, Jin R, Marikangas KR, Walters EE. Lifetime prevalence and age-of-onset distributions of DSM-IV disorders in the National Comorbidity Survey Replication. Arch Gen Psychiatry. 2005;(62):593–602. Erratum in Arch Gen Psychiatry. 2005;(62):768.
78. Davalos DB, Yadon CA, Tregellas HC. Untreated prenatal maternal depression and the potential risks to offspring: a review. Arch Womens Ment Health. 2012;15:1–14.
79. Kotch JB. Maternal and child health: programs, problems, and policy in public health. 2nd ed. Sudbury, MA: Jones and Bartlett; 2005.
80. Mohllajee AP, Curtis KM, Morrow B, Marchbanks PA. Pregnancy intention and its relationship to birth and maternal outcomes. Obstet Gynecol. 2007;109:678–86.
81. Shah PS, Balkhair T, Ohlsson A, Beyene J, Scott F, Frick C. Intention to become pregnant and low birth weight and preterm birth: a systematic review. Matern Child Health J. 2011;15:205–16.
82. Civic D, Scholes D, Ichikawa L, LaCroix AZ, Yoshida CK, Ott SM, et al. Depressive symptoms in users and non-users of depot medroxyprogesterone acetate. Contraception. 2000;61(6):385–90.
83. Westhoff C, Truman C, Kalmuss D, Cushman L, Davidson A, Rulin M, et al. Depressive symptoms and Depo-Provera®. Contraception. 1998;57(4):237–40.

84. Berenson AB, Odom SD, Breitkopf CR, Rahman M. Physiologic and psychologic symptoms associated with use of injectable contraception and 20 μg oral contraceptive pills. Am J Obstet Gynecol. 2008;199(4):351.e1–12.

85. Bartz D, Goldberg AB. Injectable contraceptives. In: Hatcher RA, Trusseull J, Nelson AL, Cates W, Kowal D, Policar MS, editors. Contraceptive technology. New York: Ardent Media, Inc.; 2011. p. 209–36.

86. Neumark-Sztainer D, Wall M, Larson NI, Eisenberg ME, Loth K. Dieting and disordered eating behaviors from adolescence to young adulthood: findings from a 10-year longitudinal study. J Am Diet Assoc. 2011;111(7):1004–11.

87. Pasternak Y, Weintraub AY, Shoham-Vardi I, Sergienko R, Guez J, Wiznitzer A, et al. Obstetric and perinatal outcomes in women with eating disorders. J Womens Health. 2012;21(1):61–5.

88. Pinkerton JV, Guico-Pabia CJ, Taylor HS. Menstrual cycle-related exacerbation of disease. Am J Obstet Gynecol. 2010;202(3): 221–31.

89. DiVasta AD, Feldman HA, Giancaterino C, Rosen CJ, LeBoff MS, Gordon CM. The effect of gonadal and adrenal steroid therapy on skeletal health in adolescents and young women with anorexia nervosa. Metabolism. 2012;61:1010–20.

90. Grinspoon S, Thomas L, Miller K, Herzog D, Klibanski A. Effects of recombinant human IGF-I and oral contraceptive administration on bone density in anorexia nervosa. J Clin Endocrinol Metab. 2002;87:2883–91.

91. Scholes D, Lacroix A, Ichikawa L, Barlow W, Ott S. Change in bone mineral density among adolescent women using and discontinuing depot medroxyprogesterone acetate contraception. Arch Pediatr Adolesc Med. 2005;159:139–44.

92. World Health Organization. Statement on hormonal contraception and bone health. Wkly Epidemiol Rec. 2005;80:302–4.

93. Lopez LM, Grimes DA, Schulz KF, Curtis KM. Steroidal contraceptives: effect on bone fractures in women. Cochrane Database Syst Rev. 2011;(7):CD006033.

94. Godart NT, Perdereau F, Rein Z, Berthoz S, Wallier J, Jeammet P, et al. Comorbidity studies of eating disorders and mood disorders: critical review of the literature. J Affect Disord. 2007;97:37–49.

95. Karceski S. Initial treatment of epilepsy in adults. UpToDate; 2013. [Updated 30 November 2012; cited 5 February 2013]. Available from: http://www.uptodate.com.

96. Christensen J, Petrenaite V, Atterman J, Sidenius P, Ohman I, Tomson T, et al. Oral contraceptives induce lamotrigine metabolism: evidence from a double-blind, placebo-controlled trial. Epilepsia. 2007;48(3):484.

Chapter 10
Adolescents with Disabilities

Sloane L. York and Cassing Hammond

WHAT IS "DISABILITY"

The first step in understanding disability is defining it. The very word "disability" conjures a range of mental images and preju- dices. Physical and mental variations, after all, are as diverse as the human condition and subject to the ever-changing influences of culture and technology.

Medical and rehabilitative models of disability traditionally have viewed disability through the prism of disease. In this context, disability arises within the individual, requires cure or treatment, and frequently results in an individual's dependence on others. Dicken's Tiny Tim, Shakespeare's Richard III, Melville's Captain Ahab, and countless other literary figures have illnesses or deformities that isolate, weaken, inspire, and empower. Even the Social Security Administration's definition of disability uses a medical/rehabilitative framework when it defines disability as "...the inability to engage in any substantial gainful activ- ity by reason of any medically determinable physical or mental impairment(s)..." [1].

Social and contextual models of disability, developed in the latter part of the twentieth century, recognize that disability often

S.L.York, M.D., M.P.H. (✉)
Department of Obstetrics and Gynecology, Rush University Medical Center,
1645 West Jackson Street, Suite 310, Chicago, IL 60612, USA
e-mail: Sloane_L_York@rush.edu

C. Hammond, M.D.
Department of Obstetrics and Gynecology, 675 North St. Claire, Suite 14-200,
Chicago, IL 60611, USA
e-mail: chammond@nmff.org

A. Whitaker and M. Gilliam (eds.), *Contraception for Adolescent and Young Adult Women*, DOI 10.1007/978-1-4614-6579-9_10,
© Springer Science + Business Media New York 2014

arises due to societal barriers—whether through architecture, communication, or negative stereotypes. The Americans with Disabilities Act (ADA) recognized that "disabled" individuals includes those whose conditions might not inherently impair their activities if reasonable public accommodations were made [2]. The World Health Organization's International Classification of Functioning, Disability and Health (ICF) similarly notes that disability "…represents a dynamic interaction between health conditions (diseases, disorders, injuries, trauma etc.) and con-textual factors" [3]. Definitions such as those used by ADA and ICF do not treat disability as a binary category that some people belong to and others do not. This "New Disability" is a con-tinuum, relevant to the lives of all people to different degrees at different times of life.

Prevalence of Disability: Reproductive Age and Women
Regardless of which model one uses to define disability, indi-viduals with disabilities comprise a growing segment of the US population—and a group more likely to interface with the health-care system [4]. According to 2010 US Census data, 56.7 million non-institutionalized persons aged 5 and older, or 18.7 % of the population, reported disability [5]. According to the American Community Survey conducted by the US Census Bureau in 2007, women age 21 and younger with disabilities comprise 8 % of the young female population [6, 7]. Many of these girls and young women require help from providers who are sensitive to their spe-cial needs as they navigate the overlooked confluence of disability, sexuality, and adolescence. A list of resources is provided to help guide patients and providers through this process (Table 10.1).

REPRODUCTIVE HEALTH: MYTHS ABOUT WOMEN WITH DISABILITIES
According to the National Organization on Disability Survey 2000, 19 % of disabled persons reported failure to obtain needed medi-cal care compared with only 7 % of those without disabilities [8]. A survey conducted by the Center for Research on Women with Disabilities reported that one-third of women with disabilities were denied care by a primary care medical office on the basis of disability [9]. Among disabled women who had given birth, roughly 56 % of respondents said their hospital could not accom-modate disability-specific needs [9]. Although barriers to health care include physical, communication, economic, and program-matic barriers, many of the problems that women with disabilities

TABLE 10.1 Resources on women with disabilities

The Arc	1825 K Street NW, Suite 1200, Washington, DC 20006, Phone: 202-534-3700, 800-433-5255, Fax: 202-534-3731	http://www.thearc.org/ E-mail: info@thearc.org
Center for Research on Women with Disabilities Baylor College of Medicine(CROWD)	One Baylor Plaza Houston, TX 77030, Phone: 800-44-CROWD (800-443-7693), 713-798-5782	http://www.bcm.edu/crowd/
Disabled Women on the Web		http://www.disabilityhistory.org/dwa/ E-mail: info@disabledwomen.net
The National Organization on Disability	5 East 86th Street New York, NY 10028, 646-505-1191, 202-293-596	http://nod.org/ E-mail: info@nod.org
Project Genesis	720 Main Street, 3rd Floor, P.O. Box 799, Willimantic, CT 06226-0799	http://www.projectgenesis.us/
Sexual Health: Expert Medical Care on Demand: Disabilities and Chronic Conditions	1.855.SEX.HEALTH (739.4325)	http://www.sexualhealth.com/ disabilities-chronic-conditions/

(continued)

TABLE 10.1 (continued)

SPINALCORD Injury Information Network	529 Spain Rehab Center 1717 6TH Ave South Birmingham, AL 35233, Phone: 205-934-3283 Fax: 205-975-4691, TDD: 205-934-4642	http://www.uab.edu/medicine/sci/ E-mail: sciweb@uab.edu
WomensHealth.gov—The Federal Source for Women's Health Information	Voice: (800) 994-9662, TDD: (888) 220-5446	http://www.womenshealth.gov/wwd/

Video or Book Resources:

Health Care Tool Kit…for individuals with disabilities and the people who support them. Wisconsin Council on Developmental Disabilities, PO Box 7851, Madison, WI 53707. Voice: (608)266-7826; TDD: (608)266-6660; Fax: (608)267-3906 http://www.wi-bpdd.org/publications/2010/Health%20Care%20Tool%20Kit%20Web.pdf

Let's Talk About Health: What Every Woman Should Know. Heaton, C, Roberts, BS, Murphy, L, Meagher, M, Randall, D. The Arc of New Jersey, Women's Health Project, 985 Livingston Ave., North Brunswick, NJ, 08902. Phone: 732-246-2525, Ext. 28 *Email: info@arcnj.org*

The Gyn Exam. Handbook: http://www.stanfield.com/products/family-life-relationships/other-family-ed-programs/ James Stanfield Co, Inc., P.O. Box 41058, Santa Barbara, CA 93140, phone: 800-421-6534

Reproductive Health for Women with Spinal Cord Injury Part 1: The Gynecological Examination. UAB Medical Rehabilitation Research and Training Center in Secondary Complications in Spinal Cord Injury. Phone: (205) 934-3283 Video accessible at *http://www.uab.edu/medicine/sci/uab-scims-information/reproductive-health-for-women-with-spinal-cord-injury-video-series*

encounter when seeking reproductive health care derive from myths shared by both lay people and health-care professionals:

- Myth 1: Disabled women are asexual and not at risk for sexually transmitted infection or pregnancy.
- Myth 2: Only independently functioning disabled women can handle sexual relationships. When disabled women have a partner, they should be especially grateful.
- Myth 3: Disabled women cannot become mothers. Either the risks of pregnancy pose too much hazard to the patient's health or the disabled mother's disability deems her unfit to parent.
- Myth 4: Common modes of contraception pose excessive risk to many women with disabilities, particularly those suffering from severe cognitive or mobility impairment.

Like most myths, several of these misperceptions persist because they contain half-truths and overgeneralizations. Some severely impaired adolescents are sexually inactive and needlessly pressured by well-intentioned caregivers to undergo pelvic exam-based screenings. Some severely disabled women do encounter problems with relationships. Indeed, women with disabilities are less likely to be married than women without disabilities, more likely to become divorced after acquiring a disability, and have lower educational attainment than women lacking disability [6]. But many women with disabilities want to parent and do parent effectively, just as other women with disabilities wish to avoid pregnancy utilizing whatever means of contraception best suits their special circumstances.

Girls with disabilities may begin to encounter misperceptions about reproduction at menarche. Even normal menstrual function can raise anxiety about menstrual hygiene, and girls restricted to wheelchairs might reasonably need assistance limiting menstrual flow. Parents also voice concerns regarding how physical maturation will further impact mobility, vulnerability to sexual abuse, and the risks that attend sexual activity including sexually transmitted infection and pregnancy [10]. Some parents request surgical sterilization, hysterectomy, or other surgeries in an attempt to prevent untoward effects of sexual maturation [11, 12].

Unfortunately, girls with disabilities often enter adolescence lacking access to reproductive health information, despite their common participation in sexual relationships and nearly twice the risk of sexual abuse compared to nondisabled peers [13]. Disabled students in grades 9–12 typically describe their health care as "fair" or "poor," suggesting that they fail to receive information and care they deem necessary [14]. Parents, the most frequent source of sexual information for children, less frequently talk about sex to disabled girls as they do with nondisabled siblings [15]. Girls with cognitive disabilities or disabilities that impair communication might have even greater difficulty. Valuable resources include the video and workbook "Let's Talk About Health: What Every Woman Should Know" designed for girls with developmental disabilities [16]. It is very important that girls and adolescents with disabilities encounter health-care professionals able to provide culturally competent disability care.

SEXUAL BEHAVIORS OF DISABLED ADOLESCENTS IN THE UNITED STATES

To provide culturally competent reproductive health care to disabled adolescents, health-care providers must understand the interplay between sexual behavior and disability. Although many providers assume severely immobilized or cognitively impaired adolescents are asexual, several data sets refute this assumption [17, 18]. In the National Longitudinal Study of Adolescent Health (Add Health), the largest US survey, Cheng and Udry [19] evaluated a nested sample of more than 900 physically disabled adolescents. The authors examined four major aspects of disabled adolescent sexual behavior: attitudes toward premarital sex, pregnancy, and birth control; school sex education exposure and birth control knowledge; friendship networks and popularity among peers; and romantic sexual attraction and coital sexual behaviors. Disabled adolescents engaged in sexual activity as frequently as nondisabled peers. Indeed, degree of mobility impairment failed to predict likelihood of sexual activity. Disabled adolescents reported higher rates of isolation, particularly from peers. Physically disabled girls had no significant difference in either knowledge or confidence in knowledge of birth control than nondisabled peers. Many disabled female adolescents viewed pregnancy and teenage pregnancy more favorably than nondisabled peers. Finally, the authors utilized multinomial logistic regression to model intercourse experiences by degree of disability, controlling for age, pubertal development, race, and family structure. Among both boys and girls, as age increases, the odds for having consensual or forced sex also increase. Although even mildly disabled girls had higher odds for consensual sex than nondisabled girls, all girls with disabilities confronted more than twice the risk of forced sex as nondisabled girls.

Disabled adolescents are a sexually "at-risk" population— at risk for unintended pregnancy, sexually transmitted infection, and forced sex. Health-care professionals need to provide comprehensive reproductive health counseling and to do so in an environment that removes some of the physical and communication barriers that so often encumber health-care encounters. As with all adolescents, adolescents with disabilities need reassurance of privacy, and they need conversations conducted without caregivers and parents present. Girls with disabilities require information regarding contraception that will help them choose a method that is medically safe and practical. Although limited studies evaluate the safety and efficacy of contraception among women with disabilities, certain common issues warrant special mention.

SPECIAL CONSIDERATIONS

Adolescents with disabilities include a diverse population of young women with both cognitive and physical limitations. Providers must tailor contraceptive regimens to the individual patient, taking into account how the contraceptive might impact the patient's disability and how the patient's disability might impact her contraceptive regimen. Limited data exists to guide clinicians in choosing the optimal contraceptive for disabled patients.

Communication

Although providers should discuss options fully with the patient, some disabilities impede communication or comprehension of information. Communication disorders range widely and are one of the most common disabilities in the United States [20, 21]. For those young women with severe cognitive and communication disabilities, providers must often rely on reports and requests from family members and personal care attendants. Generally, providers should avoid use of surrogate decision makers among cognitively intact patients including close family members [22]. Patient's who appear "globally incompetent" might only be "operationally incompetent" in that their ability to comprehend information is compensated through the use of various communication modalities [23]. Providers should remain mindful of the provider's primary obligation to the patient and consult professionals accustomed to assessing competency to avoid inadvertent discrimination against the cognitively unimpaired patient with a communication disorder [24]. Many physical medicine and rehabilitation specialists have specialized expertise to help overcome communication barriers. Indeed, fellowship training programs exist to help bolster these skills in physical medicine and rehabilitation specialists [25]. Informed consent is necessary for every patient, including women with disabilities. All patients, and/or their caregivers, should receive reasonable communication despite communication difficulties [26–28].

The Physical Exam

Physical exams may be difficult for disabled patients due to spasticity, pelvic floor atrophy, autonomic dysreflexia (AD), or a variety of other complicating issues [29]. Fortunately, an exam is not necessary to safely prescribe oral contraceptives, injectables, or implants [30]. Several simple office modifications facilitate pelvic exam, assuring patient comfort and safety. Adjustable tables that descend to wheelchair height, particularly tables equipped with side rails or handles, improve patient access [31]. Positioning patients for a pelvic exam may require alternative stirrups for those with limited mobility of their legs. Providers may need to alter the usual lithotomy positioning for a pelvic exam and, instead, have assistants support the patient's legs or place the woman in knee-chest position [29]. Moving the legs of those with contractures or muscle spasticity should be done slowly and with help to ease the patient into a position. Patients with spinal cord injuries at or above T6 are more likely to have AD during pelvic exams. To decrease the likelihood of dysreflexia, clinicians should have patients identify common triggers for AD, since these often vary among patients. She should also perform her customary bowel and bladder regimens prior to the exam, both to reduce the risk of AD and to facilitate exam [31]. Clinicians must also have latex-free products available in their offices, especially as those patients with spina bifida have a higher incidence of latex sensitivity and allergy [32].

Other Considerations

Specific concerns may need to be addressed depending on the type of disability. Many immobilized patients have hygienic problems related to menstrual flow, particularly those who already suffer from decubitus ulcers. Caregivers then may request hormonal contraception for menstrual suppression for hygiene concerns along with their contraceptive use [33].

Before initiating a contraceptive method, the provider also needs to consider how women with cognitive or physical disabilities will be able to use the method. For example, daily pill taking may be difficult for those unable to swallow, or placement of the vaginal ring may be a challenge for patients lacking manual dexterity or suffering from substantial denervation atrophy of the pelvic floor. Additionally, many women with disabilities have coexisting medical conditions that require use of medications that interact with estrogen and progestins. The interactions between medications should be reviewed in these patients and addressed as appropriate.

CONTRACEPTIVE OPTIONS
Combined Hormonal Contraceptives: Pills, Transdermal Patch, and Vaginal Ring

Combined hormonal contraceptives, which contain both estrogen (in the form of ethinyl estradiol) and a progestin, are available as pills, transdermal patches, and vaginal rings. In addition to preventing pregnancy, combination regimens offer many non-contraceptive benefits for patients with disabilities. Combined hormonal methods decrease both menstrual flow and dysmenorrhea [34]. Additionally, some women with cognitive disabilities have mood changes around the time of menses. Suppression of menses through extended cycle regimens may improve these changes in mood and decrease menstrual bleeding [33, 35].

Unfortunately many of these methods require that patients take a daily pill, apply a patch each week, or leave a vaginal ring in place for an extended time period. This challenges many patients—but particularly challenges patients with physical and cognitive disabilities. Chewable oral contraceptive pills are available for those patients who are unable to swallow or use gastric tubes for nutrition (e.g., Femcon Fe, or Generess Fe) [36]. Or pills can also be crushed and mixed with a low-residue diet. Pills can also be absorbed through the vaginal mucosa and can be placed per vagina for effective use [37]. Placement of the patch in a cognitively impaired woman may also be a challenge. Some women will attempt to remove the patch if placed on the lower abdomen, arm, or buttock. This has prompted some caregivers to apply to the upper back. Similarly, many women lack manual dexterity necessary to place or monitor placement of the vaginal ring but find that partners and personal care attendants can do so. Women with spinal cord injury also develop substantial relaxation of the pelvic floor, raising concerns regarding ring retention.

Because estrogen increases the risk of venous thromboembolism (VTE), many clinicians question the advisability of prescribing estrogen-containing regimens to patients whose risk of VTE might already be increased due to immobility. Although immobility likely increases the risk of VTE, the extent to which differing degrees of immobilization quantifiably increase such risk remains unclear. The extent to which transfers and other activities prescribed for chronically immobilized patients offset the risk of VTE is also unclear. Certainly, pregnancy exposes patients to a greater risk of VTE than any combination contraception regimen. Neither the World Health Organization (WHO) nor the American Congress of Obstetricians and Gynecologists (ACOG) limit the use of estrogen-containing products in immobilized patients [36, 38].

However, most clinicians minimize estrogen dose and become more reluctant to prescribe estrogen with increasing degrees of immobility—particularly among patients who might have a reasonable alternative. When examining the pharmacokinetics of each combined methods, the patch exposes patients to 3.4 times more estrogen than the vaginal ring and 1.6 times more than oral contraceptives with 30 μg of ethinyl estradiol and 150 μg levonorgestrel [39]. Many providers avoid the patch or similarly estrogenic regimens among completely immobilized patients such as quadriplegics.

A number of women with disabilities also have seizures and may be on antiepileptic drugs (AEDs). The efficacy of estrogen-containing products or the efficacy of AEDs may be altered through the use of both products [40]. The clinician should review what interactions may occur and work in tandem with the patient's neurologist to make sure the patient has appropriate seizure control and contraception. Centers for Disease Control and Prevention's US Medical Eligibility Criteria (MEC) for Contraceptive Use [41], which represent a consensus opinion of experts in family planning and disease management based on the current literature, give the following medications a Category 3 recommendation (risks outweigh benefits) for estrogen-containing contraceptives: lamotrigine (as monotherapy), phenytoin, carbamazepine, barbiturates, primidone, topiramate, and oxcarbazepine. See Table 9.1 of Chap. 9 "Women and Girls with Medical Illness" for more details on the interaction between AEDs and hormonal contraception.

Progestin-Only Methods: Pills, Injectables, and Implants
Progestin-only methods of contraception provide many of the contraceptive and non-contraceptive benefits desired by individuals with disabilities but avoid VTE risk associated with estrogen. A number of progestin-only products are available including progestin-only pills (POPs), depot medroxyprogesterone acetate (DMPA), and contraceptive implants. Progestin-only methods do not significantly increase the risk of venous or arterial thromboembolism, including stroke or myocardial infarction, and may be used in women who may be at increased risk of thrombosis, like those who have limited mobility.

Most POPs used in the United States contain norethindrone or norgestrel in doses that modify the endometrium and cervical mucus without consistent inhibition of ovulation [42]. Long-term use may lead to amenorrhea in 10–20 % of women, but many have irregular bleeding [36, 42]. The irregular bleeding is a large reason for discontinuation [43] and may be a hygiene issue for some disabled women.

DMPA is an injectable contraceptive that offers many advantages to adolescents and the disabled. Two methods of administration are approved in the United States which are equally effective contraceptives: 150 mg injected intramuscularly and 104 mg injected subcutaneously [44]. Currently, both are approved for administration by health-care providers, but a number of recent studies have examined the safety and acceptability of self-administration of subcutaneous DMPA, which would potentially be easier for caregivers of some disabled women [45, 46].

Up to 70 % of women experience irregular bleeding with DMPA, but over time this improves and eventually most are amenorrheic [42]. Up to 46–70 % of DMPA users may be amenorrheic after 12 months of use [42, 47–49]. Many adolescents with disabilities have used DMPA due to the favorable bleeding profile and the subsequent improved hygiene. One small study suggested that DMPA improved cyclic behavioral changes among cognitively disabled women [50]. Some have questioned the relationship between DMPA use and depression. The results are mixed with some studies noting an association [51], while others report insignificant results [52, 53]. Specifically among adolescents using DMPA, one study did not find any hormonal changes [53]. The implications for those disabled adolescents with mood disorders are unknown. The US MEC gives all methods of contraception a Category 1 (no restrictions on use) for women with depressive disorders [41]. Also see Chap. 9.

DMPA use is equally efficacious in obese women as in normal weight women [42]. While weight gain is not significant with most DMPA users, recent research has recognized that some women are more susceptible to weight gain [54, 55]. This is particularly worrisome among disabled patients already at risk for weight gain due to immobilization and whose weight gain might complicate transfers. See Chap. 8, "Contraception for Women and Girls Who Are Obese," for more detail on the relationship between DMPA and weight gain.

DMPA is associated with a reduction in bone mineral density that is reversible and not associated with long-term fracture risk among the general population. Despite the 2004 warning from the US Food and Drug Administration (FDA) for these concerns, ACOG does not recommend stopping DMPA or checking BMD in healthy patients. See Chap. 4 "Progestin-Only Contraception" for detailed discussion of DMPA and BMD in healthy women. When confronted with immobilized patients, or others who have an increased risk of osteopenia or osteoporosis, long-term use of DMPA may cause significant bone loss. Watson et al. [56] report that use of DMPA by women of all ages with developmental disabilities results in an increase risk of osteoporotic fractures with an odds ratio of 2.4. This result was based on 13 fractures in 340 DMPA users from a non-institutionalized population. Additionally, Arvio et al. [57] reported a decreased BMD and an increase in fracture rates among 51 cognitively disabled, institutionalized women (pre- and postmenopausal) when compared to controls. No study specifically has examined DMPA use in disabled adolescents, and it is difficult to extrapolate data from nondisabled adolescents or from disabled adults to this population.

Implanon, Jadelle, and Norplant are the three contraceptive implants available around the world, though in the United States, only Implanon, a single-rod etonogestrel (ENG) implant, is available. The ENG implant is a three-year implant and is a highly effective form of contraception that may be appropriate for many disabled adolescents. The levels of etonogestrel suppress ovulation, potentially improving dysmenorrhea or endometriosis [58]. Unfortunately, relatively high rates of irregular bleeding may hinder its use among some immobilized patients. Use of this implant does not appear to impact BMD [59].

Few medications impair the contraceptive efficacy of progestin-only methods with the exception of some antiepileptic drugs (AEDs). Carbamazepine and other enzyme-inducing medications increases metabolism of the ENG in the ENG implant and pregnancy has been reported in association with this [60]. However, the US MEC gives the etonogestrel implant a Category 2 (benefits outweigh risks) for the following AEDs: phenytoin, carbamazepine, barbiturates, primidone, topiramate, and oxcarbazepine [41]. Additionally, AEDs may increase bone loss. If using certain AEDs and DMPA concurrently, especially if DMPA is given at higher doses, it is uncertain how this may affect BMD.

Intrauterine Devices
Two intrauterine devices (IUD) are currently available in the United States: a levonorgestrel IUD (Mirena®) and a copper IUD (Paragard®). The copper IUD is approved for nulliparous patients including adolescents and this extends to disabled adolescents. The package labeling for the levonorgestrel IUD (LNG-IUD) states that it is recommend for women with at least one child, but both ACOG and the Society for Family Planning find this an acceptable method of contraception in nulliparous women [61, 62]. The US MEC give a Category 2 (benefits outweigh risks) for nulliparous patients. Both are highly effective contraceptives, preventing pregnancy in >99 %.

The LNG-IUD has the additional benefit of decreasing menstrual flow by 40–50 % and approximately one-third of women becoming amenorrheic [42, 63]. Additionally, this IUD has been demonstrated to improve dysmenorrhea [63]. Pillai et al. [64] published a small case series looking at the use of the LNG-IUD in disabled adolescents and found high acceptability and satisfaction (in 13 of 14 women who used the method), along with a reduction in menorrhagia. The copper IUD is an excellent form of contraception but will neither suppress menstruation nor improve dysmenorrhea.

Placement of an IUD could potentially be difficult for adolescents with disabilities. Physical disabilities may limit patient positioning for placement. Women with cognitive disabilities may not cooperate easily with a pelvic exam. In some circumstances, a patient may require sedation to tolerate placement of an IUD, and this may be more common among women and girls with physical and cognitive disabilities. The risks and benefits of sedation must be weighed against the potential long-term benefits of IUD placement.

Some clinicians are concerned about placing IUDs in patients with limited abilities to sense lower abdominal pain or other signs of infections, perforation, or expulsion. Given the generally low risk for all complication other than spontaneous expulsion, these concerns are unwarranted. Women with spinal cord injuries who have use of their upper extremities may check the IUD strings to confirm expulsion or perforation has not occurred. Those who have less manual dexterity may have their partner checked for IUD strings or returned for confirmation of correct placement 4–6weeks after insertion. Finally, as with other methods that induce amenorrhea, the LNG-IUD offers spinal cord injury patients an opportunity to prevent menstrual-related dysreflexia without the fear of weight gain and bone loss related to DMPA.

Emergency Contraception

A number of options exist for emergency contraception (EC) in the United States including the copper IUD, 150 mg of levonorgestrel (Plan B), and ulipristal (Ella). EC should not be withheld from an adolescent with any disability. All adolescents—including adolescents with disabilities—should have access to EC when needed. Levonorgestrel pills have no risk of thrombosis and so can be used in immobilized patients or other patients at risk of thrombosis without concern. These pills are available over the counter for women over 17 years of age or by prescription for those younger. Recently approved by the FDA, ulipristal is available by prescription. See Chap. 6 "Emergency Contraception" for a thorough overall discussion of EC for adolescents.

Barrier Methods

Barrier methods are user dependent and therefore rely upon the woman or man using the contraceptive during intercourse. For some women with disabilities, placement of any of these methods may be difficult to achieve physically or, for some of those with cognitive impairments, may be difficult to understand how to use the method. A number of women may have partners who can help with placement. Male condoms are dependent upon the male partner and so may be a good option for some women with motivated partners. Latex-free methods should be recommended to those women with spina bifida who may be at high risk of latex sensitivity or allergy. See Chap. 2 "Barrier Methods" for a thorough overall discussion of barrier methods for adolescents.

Sterilization

Parents or caregivers may broach the topic of sterilization as a young woman enters puberty. Often they are concerned with more than just prevention of pregnancy—concerns about menstrual hygiene and issues surrounding sexual maturation may predominate. Sterilization for young women with cognitive or developmental disabilities has been an area of significant concern as many young women underwent forced sterilization in the past. It is key to assess the young woman's decision-making capabilities and determine if she is competent to consent [65]. If she is judged unable to consent but her parent or guardian is requesting this, the physician and surgeon must fully evaluate the circumstances of her disability and comorbidities. A developmental or cognitive disability alone is not a justified reason for permanent sterilization [65].

Beyond sterilization, some caregivers have requested hysterectomies to stop menstruation and potentially the pubertal process if oophorectomy was to be performed. In the past this has been granted in specific cases. Performing either sterilization or hysterectomy on a young woman without the ability to consent for herself is potentially ethically questionable and must be fully reviewed. The case of Ashley X [11] generated a lot of controversy when a girl with static encephalopathy had a hysterectomy and resection of breast buds at age of 6 [66]. Each case is entirely individual and, like this case, the risks and benefits, along with the long-term consequences, must be balanced. For a woman with very different circumstances, Stainton [10] writes of her own sterilization during her teen years and her long-time regret of undergoing a hysterectomy because she did not have the opportunity to parent. Both cases are unique, but not entirely different to what women with disabilities and their caregivers may consider. As a health-care provider, the patient's best interests must always be considered when developing a plan that will have long-term consequences, like sterilization.

SUMMARY

A number of contraceptive options exist that are long acting and highly efficacious and many with the added benefit of menstrual control in the case of the levonorgestrel IUD, implants, or injectables. Of course, long-term treatment with a contraceptive must be fully evaluated when caring for adolescents with disabilities. The clinician who cares for these young women have a unique and important job of advocating on behalf of their patients, sometimes even to parents or others who care very much of the young woman.

REFERENCES

1. Disability evaluation under social security. Social security online. 2008. http://www.ssa.gov/disability/professionals/bluebook/general-info.htm. Accessed 23 Mar 2012.
2. American with Disabilities Act of 1990. 2009. http://www.ada.gov/pubs/adastatute08.htm. Accessed 8 Mar 2014.
3. World Health Organization. International classification of functioning, disability and health. Geneva: World Health Organization; 2001.
4. Dejong G, Palsbo SE, Beatty PW, Jones GC, Knoll T, Neri MT. The organization and financing of health services for persons with disabilities. Milbank Q. 2002;80:261–301.
5. Brault MW. Americans with disabilities: 2010. Current Population Reports, July 2010. p. 1–24.
6. Kirschner KL, P RJ, Mukherjee D, Hammond C. Empowering women with disabilities to be self-determining in their health care. In: Frontera WR, Gans BM, Walsh NE, Robinson LR, eds. DeLisa's physical medicine and rehabilitation: principles and practice. 5 ed. Philadelphia: Lippincott Williams & Wilkins; 2010.
7. Jans L, Stoddard S. Chartbook on women and disability in the United States. U.S. Department of Education: Washington, DC; 1999.
8. Executive summary: 2000N.O.D./Harris survey of Americans with disabilities. National Organization on Disability. 2011. http://nod.org/research_publications/nod_harris_survey/2000_survey_of_americans_with_disabilities/. Accessed 23 Mar 2012.
9. National study on women with physical disabilities: final report 1992–1996. Baylor College of Medicine: Center for Research on

Women with Disabilities. 2009. http://www.bcm.edu/crowd/index. cfm?pmid=1408—hc. Accessed 23 Mar 2012.

10. Stainton M. A piece of my mind. Raising a woman. JAMA. 2006; 296:1445–6.

11. Gunther DF, Diekema DS. Attenuating growth in children with profound developmental disability: a new approach to an old dilemma. Arch Pediatr Adolesc Med. 2006;160:1013–7.

12. Kirschner KL, Brashler R, Savage TA. Ashley X. Am J Phys Med Rehabil. 2007;86:1023–9.

13. Murphy NA, Elias ER. Sexuality of children and adolescents with developmental disabilities. Pediatrics. 2006;118:398–403.

14. Everett Jones S, Lollar DJ. Relationship between physical disabilities or long-term health problems and health risk behaviors or conditions among US high school students. J Sch Health. 2008; 78:252–7. quiz 98–9.

15. Rousso H. Sexuality and a positive sense of self. In: Krotoski DM, Nosek MA, Turk MA, editors. Women with physical disabilities: achieving and maintaining health and well-being. Baltimore, MD: Brookes; 1996. p. 109–16.

16. Heaton C, Roberts BS, Murphy L. Let's talk about health: what every woman should know. The Arc of New Jersey: North Brunswick, NJ; 1996.

17. Choquet M, Du Pasquier FL, Manfredi R. Sexual behavior among adolescents reporting chronic conditions: a French national survey. J Adolesc Health. 1997;20:62–7.

18. Suris JC, Resnick MD, Cassuto N, Blum RW. Sexual behavior of adolescents with chronic disease and disability. J Adolesc Health. 1996;19:124–31.

19. Cheng MM, Udry JR. Sexual behaviors of physically disabled adolescents in the United States. J Adolesc Health. 2002;31:48–58.

20. Incidence and prevalence of communication disorders and hearing loss in children—2008 edition. American Speech-Language-Hearing Association. 2012. http://www.asha.org/research/reports/ children.htm. Accessed 2 Dec 2012.

21. Incidence and prevalence of speech, voice, and language disorders in adults in the United States: 2008 edition. American Speech-Language-Hearing Association. 2012. http://www.asha.org/ Research/reports/speech_voice_language/. Accessed 2 Dec 2012.

22. Kagan A, Kimelman MDZ. Informed consent in aphasia research: myth or reality. Clin Aphasiol. 1995;23:65–75.

23. Alexander MP. Clinical determination of mental competence. A theory and a retrospective study. Arch Neurol. 1988;45:23–6.

24. Leo RJ. Competency and the capacity to make treatment decisions: a primer for primary care physicians. Prim Care Companion J Clin Psychiatry. 1999;1:131–41.

25. Advanced rehabilitation training: interventions for neurologic communication disorders. Northwestern University Feinberg School of Medicine. 2012. http://www.feinberg.northwestern.edu/

sites/pmr/education/research-fellowships/AdvancedRehabilitation Training.html. Accessed 4 Dec 2012.

26. ACOG Committee on Ethics. ACOG Committee Opinion No. 439: Informed consent. Obstet Gynecol. 2009;114:401–8.

27. Informed consent, parental permission, and assent in pediatric practice. Committee on Bioethics. J Child Fam Nurs. 1998;(1): 57–61.

28. Pediatric Decision Making. American Medical Association. 2010. http://www.ama-assn.org/resources/doc/code-medical-ethics/10016a.pdf, http://www.ama-assn.org/resources/doc/code-medical-ethics/10016b.pdf. Accessed 2 Dec 2012.

29. Kaplan C. Special issues in contraception: caring for women with disabilities. J Midwifery Womens Health. 2006;51:450–6.

30. Stewart FH, Harper CC, Ellertson CE, Grimes DA, Sawaya GF, Trussell J. Clinical breast and pelvic examination requirements for hormonal contraception: current practice vs evidence. JAMA. 2001;285:2232–9.

31. Welner SL, Foley CC, Nosek MA, Holmes A. Practical considerations in the performance of physical examinations on women with disabilities. Obstet Gynecol Surv. 1999;54:457–62.

32. Buck D, Michael T, Wahn U, Niggemann B. Ventricular shunts and the prevalence of sensitization and clinically relevant allergy to latex in patients with spina bifida. Pediatr Allergy Immunol. 2000; 11:111–5.

33. Savasi I, Spitzer RF, Allen LM, Ornstein MP. Menstrual suppression for adolescents with developmental disabilities. J Pediatr Adolesc Gynecol. 2009;22:143–9.

34. Kiley J, Hammond C. Combined oral contraceptives: a comprehensive review. Clin Obstet Gynecol. 2007;50:868–77.

35. Quint EH, Breech L, Bacon J, Schwandt A. Management quandary. Menstrual issues in a teenager with developmental delay. J Pediatr Adolesc Gynecol. 2006;19:53–5.

36. American College of Obstetricians and Gynecologists Committee on Adolescent Health Care. ACOG Committee Opinion No. 448: menstrual manipulation for adolescents with disabilities. Obstet Gynecol. 2009;114:1428–31.

37. Coutinho EM, da Silva AR, Carreira C, Rodrigues V, Goncalves MT. Conception control by vaginal administration of pills containing ethinyl estradiol and dl-norgestrel. Fertil Steril. 1984;42:478–81.

38. World Health Organization. Medical eligibility criteria for contraceptive use. 4th ed. Geneva: World Health Organization; 2010.

39. van den Heuvel MW, van Bragt AJ, Alnabawy AK, Kaptein MC. Comparison of ethinylestradiol pharmacokinetics in three hormonal contraceptive formulations: the vaginal ring, the transdermal patch and an oral contraceptive. Contraception. 2005;72:168–74.

40. Dutton C, Foldvary-Schaefer N. Contraception in women with epilepsy: pharmacokinetic interactions, contraceptive options, and management. Int Rev Neurobiol. 2008;83:113–34.

41. Centers for Disease Control and Prevention (CDC). U.S. Medical Eligibility Criteria for Contraceptive Use, 2010. MMWR Recomm Rep. 2010;59:1–86.
42. Speroff L, Darney PD. A clinical guide for contraception. 5th ed. Philadelphia: Wolters Kluwer Health/Lippincott Williams & Wilkins; 2011.
43. Broome M, Fotherby K. Clinical experience with the progestogen-only pill. Contraception. 1990;42:489–95.
44. Simon MA, Shulman LP. Subcutaneous versus intramuscular depot methoxyprogesterone acetate: a comparative review. Womens Health (Lond Engl). 2006;2:191–7.
45. Cameron ST, Glasier A, Johnstone A. Pilot study of home self-administration of subcutaneous depo-medroxyprogesterone acetate for contraception. Contraception. 2011;85(5):458–64.
46. Prabhakaran S, Sweet A. Self-administration of subcutaneous depot medroxyprogesterone acetate for contraception: feasibility and acceptability. Contraception. 2011;85(5):453–7.
47. Arias RD, Jain JK, Brucker C, Ross D, Ray A. Changes in bleeding patterns with depot medroxyprogesterone acetate subcutaneous injection 104mg. Contraception. 2006;74:234–8.
48. Sangi-Haghpeykar H, Poindexter 3rd AN, Bateman L, Ditmore JR. Experiences of injectable contraceptive users in an urban setting. Obstet Gynecol. 1996;88:227–33.
49. Westhoff C. Depot-medroxyprogesterone acetate injection (Depo-Provera): a highly effective contraceptive option with proven long-term safety. Contraception. 2003;68:75–87.
50. Quint EH. Gynecological health care for adolescents with developmental disabilities. Adolesc Med. 1999;(10):221–9, vi.
51. Civic D, Scholes D, Ichikawa L, et al. Depressive symptoms in users and non-users of depot medroxyprogesterone acetate. Contraception. 2000;61:385–90.
52. Kaunitz AM. Long-acting hormonal contraception: assessing impact on bone density, weight, and mood. Int J Fertil Womens Med. 1999;44:110–7.
53. Gupta N, O'Brien R, Jacobsen LJ, et al. Mood changes in adolescents using depot-medroxyprogesterone acetate for contraception: a prospective study. J Pediatr Adolesc Gynecol. 2001;14:71–6.
54. Kaneshiro B, Edelman A. Contraceptive considerations in overweight teens. Curr Opin Obstet Gynecol. 2011;23:344–9.
55. Bonny AE, Ziegler J, Harvey R, Debanne SM, Secic M, Cromer BA. Weight gain in obese and nonobese adolescent girls initiating depot medroxyprogesterone, oral contraceptive pills, or no hormonal contraceptive method. Arch Pediatr Adolesc Med. 2006;160:40–5.
56. Watson KC, Lentz MJ, Cain KC. Associations between fracture incidence and use of depot medroxyprogesterone acetate and anti-epileptic drugs in women with developmental disabilities. Womens Health Issues. 2006;16:346–52.

57. Arvio M, Kilpinen-Loisa P, Tiitinen A, Huovinen K, Makitie O. Bone mineral density and sex hormone status in intellectually disabled women on progestin-induced amenorrhea. Acta Obstet Gynecol Scand. 2009;88:428–33.
58. Walch K, Unfried G, Huber J, et al. Implanon versus medroxyprogesterone acetate: effects on pain scores in patients with symptomatic endometriosis–a pilot study. Contraception. 2009;79:29–34.
59. Beerthuizen R, van Beek A, Massai R, Makarainen L, Hout J, Bennink HC. Bone mineral density during long-term use of the progestogen contraceptive implant Implanon compared to a non-hormonal method of contraception. Hum Reprod. 2000;15: 118–22.
60. Schindlbeck C, Janni W, Friese K. Failure of Implanon contraception in a patient taking carbamazepine for epilepsia. Arch Gynecol Obstet. 2006;273:255–6.
61. Lyus R, Lohr P, Prager S, Board of the Society of Family Planning. Use of the Mirena LBG-IUS and Paragard CuT380A intrauterine devices in nulliparous women, SFP guideline 20092. Contraception. 2010;81:367–71.
62. Deans EI, Grimes DA. Intrauterine devices for adolescents: a systematic review. Contraception. 2009;79:418–23.
63. Bednarek PH, Jensen JT. Safety, efficacy and patient acceptability of the contraceptive and non-contraceptive uses of the LNG-IUD. Int J Womens Health. 2010;1:45–58.
64. Pillai M, O'Brien K, Hill E. The levonorgestrel intrauterine system (Mirena) for the treatment of menstrual problems in adolescents with medical disorders, or physical or learning disabilities. BJOG. 2010;117:216–21.
65. Sterilization of minors with developmental disabilities. American Academy of Pediatrics. Committee on Bioethics. Pediatrics. 1999; (104):337–40.
66. Diekema DS, Fost N. Ashley revisited: a response to the critics. Am J Bioeth. 2010;10:30–44.

Chapter 11
Postpartum Contraception for Adolescents

Juliana Melo and Stephanie Teal

INTRODUCTION

Adolescent mothers are more likely to experience a repeat pregnancy prior to the age of 20 than other adolescent women are to become pregnant a single time [1–4]. American teens who have delivered have a 12–44 % risk of pregnancy within the first 12 months after birth [5]. This high rate of repeat pregnancy is associated with poor maternal and fetal outcomes, lack of continuing education, unemployment, and poverty [6, 7]. Characteristics associated with repeat adolescent pregnancy include both non-modifiable factors, such as minority race or ethnicity, family poverty, and young maternal age at first birth (<16 years), and modifiable factors, such as school continuation, depression or stress, and no future-oriented plans [8]. A variety of factors influence adolescent postpartum usage of contraception. In this chapter, we will review issues particularly relevant to contraceptive initiation and continuation in postpartum adolescents and young women and review the evidence regarding specific interventions.

POSTPARTUM CONSIDERATIONS

The postpartum period is one of many physical, social, and emotional changes. Many of the concerns specific to the immediate and later postpartum periods can impact contraceptive use.

J. Melo, M.D. • S. Teal, M.D., M.P.H. (✉)
Department of Obstetrics and Gynecology, University of Colorado School of Medicine, 12631 East 17th Avenue, B198-2, Aurora, CO 80045, USA
e-mail: juliana.melo@ucdenver.edu; Stephanie.Teal@ucdenver.edu

A. Whitaker and M. Gilliam (eds.), *Contraception for Adolescent and Young Adult Women*, DOI 10.1007/978-1-4614-6579-9_11,
© Springer Science + Business Media New York 2014

Body Image

Adolescence is a time of intense attention to appearance and comparison to peers. Adolescent mothers may be more likely to decline hormonal contraception for fear of weight gain or concerns about body image. The physical changes of pregnancy may be especially upsetting because they occur at a time of transition from a childish to an adult body habitus. Healthcare providers should try to elicit these concerns and address them appropriately. Patients may be reassured that combined hormonal methods (oral contraceptive pill (OCP), contraceptive transdermal patch, contraceptive vaginal ring) have not been associated with increased weight gain in users compared to nonusers [9, 10]. Additionally, no such association has been reported with the levonorgestrel intrauterine device (IUD), copper IUD, subdermal etonogestrel implant, and progestin-only pills. With regard to depot medroxyprogesterone acetate (DMPA), however, weight gain has been reported in over half of adolescents using this method and is cited as the primary reason for discontinuation by 41 % of young women in this age group [11, 12]. Interestingly, adolescents and young women who were obese at initiation of DMPA have been shown to gain significantly more weight than a similar cohort using combined OCPs or no hormonal contraceptive method [13]. These obese young women also gained more weight than all other non-obese women using DMPA [13]. While obesity is not a contraindication to the use of DMPA, a thorough discussion regarding the potential risks of worsening obesity versus the benefit of this efficacious contraceptive method is warranted in this subset of patients. [See Chap. 8: Contraception for Women and Girls Who Are Obese for further discussion.]

Sexuality and Relationships

Characteristics of adolescent sexuality, which may make consistent use of contraception difficult, may be exacerbated in young mothers. Providers who do not feel comfortable discussing teen sexuality may find themselves willing to accept a teen's statement that she has "learned her lesson" and will not need contraception any time soon. Even providers open to discussing adolescent sexuality may find that their patients are unwilling to admit that they are likely to engage in sexual behavior soon. The mental ability to move rapidly and frequently between two opposing positions, such as wanting to become pregnant and acting to remain nonpregnant, is a hallmark of the developmental stage of adolescence and exacerbates the risk of unprotected intercourse. Teens are more likely to have brief but intense relationships, which are susceptible to intercourse without contraception. Finally, teens are more likely to have periods of time without sexual activity during which they may not perceive need for continued contraception.

A frequent postpartum concern is decreased libido, which a young woman may not feel comfortable discussing with her provider and which is frequently blamed on contraceptive use. If she already perceives an unstable relationship with her baby's father, fear that successful family formation may be disrupted by further reduction in her sex drive may lead to early contraceptive discontinuation. As in all patients, unaddressed fears can lead to diminished adherence to contraceptive regimens. The status of the relationship plays an important role in contraceptive use among adolescent mothers. Established adolescent couples are less likely to consistently use contraception. In a study examining the reasons for ineffective contraceptive use among adolescents, Sheeder et al. found that participants who were not ready to try to prevent conception consistently were more likely to be living with the father of the child rather than their parents, living in a non-chaotic environment, be of Hispanic ethnicity, and have future educational/career goals that were compatible with adolescent childbearing [14]. Other studies have similarly found that young women living with their male partners were more likely to have repeat pregnancies.

Depression

Postpartum depression is common among adolescent mothers. In a 4-year prospective study following mothers age 18 and younger, over 50 % reported moderate to severe depressive symptoms [15]. Teen mothers should be routinely screened for depressive symptoms and referrals made as necessary [16]. Depression has been reported as a risk factor for rapid-repeat pregnancy [17]. This may be related to decreased contraceptive use associated with blunted motivation generally, commonly seen with depression, or specific diminished motivation to actively prevent pregnancy because pregnancy is seen as an escape from situational factors. The Centers for Disease Control and Prevention's Medical Eligibility Criteria for Contraceptive Use (USMEC) do not recommend restriction of any type of contraceptive in women with a past or current history of depression; however, data is limited [18]. (See also Chap. 9: Women and Girls with Medical Illness, section on mental illness.)

Lactation

Due to its well-documented health benefits to both mother and child, the American College of Obstetricians and Gynecologists

(ACOG) as well as the World Health Organization (WHO) recommends breastfeeding for all infants. Maternal benefits include faster recovery from childbirth, enhanced weight loss, and decreased cost. Long-term maternal benefits include reduction in breast and ovarian cancer risks [19]. Benefits to the infant include improved nutrition, host defense, and psychological well-being [19]. Long-term benefits to the infant include protection against acute illnesses and reduction in the incidence of asthma, obesity, adult cardiovascular disease, and diabetes mellitus [19]. Unfortunately, mothers under the age of 20 have the lowest rate of initiation of breastfeeding (51 %) [20]. Of those young women who initiate breastfeeding, the rate of discontinuation is rapid. Like all postpartum women, adolescent and young adult mothers should be encouraged to breastfeed their infants for as long as possible, with the goal of exclusively breastfeeding for at least 6 months.

The appropriateness of different postpartum contraceptives changes with the initiation, continuation, and frequency of breastfeeding. If the patient chooses a hormonal contraceptive while continuing to breastfeed, important aspects to consider include contraceptive effectiveness, effect of the method on milk production, and possible hormonal transfer to the infant. In pregnancy, high levels of estrogen and progesterone block the effect of prolactin on breast tissue. Full milk production does not begin until a few days after delivery, when estrogen and progesterone levels have dropped considerably. Thus, concern has long existed that giving hormonal contraceptives during lactation would diminish milk production.

A systematic review of randomized controlled trials on this topic found only five trials that compared a combined hormonal contraceptive to another hormonal contraceptive or placebo in lactating women [21]. The authors concluded that these studies were of limited quality and did not have the ability to demonstrate an effect of hormonal contraceptives on milk quantity and quality. Given the lack of high-quality evidence, many practitioners suggest waiting until milk supply and breastfeeding are well established before starting a contraceptive and using a non-hormonal or progestin-only contraceptive until weaning.

Method-specific recommendations for use during lactation are discussed below, under "method-specific considerations."

Logistical Barriers
Logistical barriers may exacerbate insufficient contraceptive use among adolescent mothers. These can include clinic and service accessibility, insurance coverage, cost of contraceptives, perceived

or real lack of confidentiality, and provider and system level biases. For instance, mothers who qualified for Medicaid coverage during pregnancy may lose contraceptive coverage after 6 weeks postpartum. Depending on the facility at which the teens receive care, some methods of contraception may not be available to them due to provider discomfort. There is still significant provider bias against IUDs for adolescents and young women regardless of parity [22, 23]. Providers often cite safety concerns regarding increased risk of STIs in this age group or fear of difficult insertion. Lack of STI testing prior to presentation for contraceptive consult is not a contraindication to IUD insertion. As long as there are no signs or symptoms of pelvic inflammatory disease, concurrent STI testing can be performed on the day of IUD insertion [24]. (See also Chap. 5: Intrauterine Devices.) Cost is another logistical barrier young women face when choosing an effective contraceptive method. If not covered by insurance, many methods can be quite costly and therefore create a barrier to initiation and consistent use. Even if a teen has insurance through her parents, privacy concerns may prevent her from using it to obtain expensive contraceptives.

METHOD-SPECIFIC CONSIDERATIONS FOR POSTPARTUM ADOLESCENTS

Contraceptive methods have been reviewed in prior chapters. In this section, we will focus specifically on method-specific considerations related to use by adolescents in the early and later postpartum periods.

Lactational amenorrhea (LAM): Non-breastfeeding women start ovulating around 4 weeks postpartum, and most women ovulate before the first menses occurs. Thus, a significant number of women are at risk for pregnancy in the immediate postpartum period. Lactational amenorrhea is an effective method of contraception within the first 6 months postpartum. It is considered over 97 % effective as long as the following criteria are met: less than 6 months postpartum, not yet resumed menses, and exclusively breastfeeding without supplementation [25–28]. This method requires a high level of motivation and commitment. Young mothers are much less likely to initiate breastfeeding than adults, and those who do breastfeed do so less frequently, with less intensity, and discontinue sooner [29, 30]. Thus, while breastfeeding should be strongly recommended to young mothers, relying on LAM for contraception should be discouraged. If a patient strongly desires to use LAM, a transition plan to a highly effective method should be discussed well in advance of when this is no longer appropriate for her.

Combined hormonal contraceptives: Combined hormonal contraceptives include estrogen and progestin: combined OCPs, the contraceptive transdermal patch, and the contraceptive vaginal ring. The risk of deep venous thromboembolism (DVT) is increased approximately fourfold throughout the pregnancy. In the immediate postpartum period, the risk is even greater, rising another five to tenfold above the baseline risk. Women must delay estrogen-containing methods until at least 21 days postpartum. Those with other risk factors for DVT should delay these methods until after 42 days postpartum.

ACOG, WHO, and the International Planned Parenthood Federation (IPPF) all advise against the use of combined hormonal contraceptives in lactating women, mostly based on the theoretical concern for decreased milk production, discussed above. In July 2011, the CDC updated its USMEC to reflect new guidance on the use of contraception in the postpartum period [31]. The updated USMEC gives a Category 2 recommendation (benefits outweigh risks) for the use of combined hormonal methods for breastfeeding women who are at least 30 days postpartum and do not have other risk factors for VTE and for all breastfeeding women greater than 42 days postpartum.

Progestin-only contraceptives: Exogenous progestins are not associated with increased risk of venous thromboembolism. Because of this, many providers recommend using progestin-only contraception until 6 weeks postpartum, after which combined hormonal methods may be resumed. Progestin-only methods, such as progestin-only pills, DMPA, or the subdermal implant, may be initiated immediately postpartum. For non-breastfeeding women, the postpartum USMEC gives a Category 1 for all progestin-only methods at any point in the postpartum period, including the etonogestrel subdermal implant, which is long-acting and highly effective and can be safely inserted in the immediate postpartum (i.e., before hospital discharge).

Studies with progestin-only contraceptives postpartum have been consistently reassuring with regard to milk production, maternal health parameters, and infant growth [32–39]. DMPA has been studied extensively in the postpartum period and found to have minimal effect on milk quality, production, and infant growth [40]. The etonogestrel subdermal implant has also been studied in the immediate postpartum period and found to have minimal effect on breastfeeding parameters and infant growth [41]. Studies on progestin-only pills, injectables, and implants initiated as soon as 2 days postpartum have found reassuring results on breastfeeding continuation, milk quality, and infant growth. For breastfeeding women, the postpartum USMEC gives these methods Category 2 at less than 30 days postpartum and Category 1 (no restrictions) for 30 days and beyond.

Intrauterine devices: Copper-bearing and levonorgestrel IUDs provide effective contraception which is long-acting, reversible, and essentially maintenance-free. These are excellent options for adolescent mothers who are motivated to avoid pregnancy. ACOG recommends long-acting reversible contraceptives as first line for all young sexually active women wishing to avoid pregnancy [42]. In breastfeeding mothers, copper-bearing IUDs do not increase breast milk copper concentration [43]. The systemic dose of levonorgestrel in the LNG-IUS is lower than that of progestin-only contraceptive pills. A randomized trial of over 300 women that compared breastfeeding performance, infant growth, and infant development over 1 year in women assigned to the Cu-IUD versus the LNG-IUS found no differences in any of these parameters [44].

When IUDs are placed in the early postpartum period, between 2 days and 6 weeks after delivery, the risk of expulsion or uterine perforation may be higher if uterine involution is not complete. Immediate postplacental IUD placement, defined as insertion within 10 min of delivery of the placenta, has been gaining popularity in the United States. Advantages include early contraceptive protection prior to resuming intercourse, no interference with breastfeeding, and an opportunity to achieve contraception for women with little access to medical care. Immediate IUD placement has not been associated with increased perforation, infection, abnormal postpartum bleeding, or uterine subinvolution. For postplacental insertion, the postpartum USMEC assigns a Category 2 for the LNG-IUS and a Category 1 for the copper IUD. Both IUDs are given a Category 2 for insertion between 10 min to 4 weeks after delivery and Category 1 beyond 4 weeks.

Promoting Contraceptive Success
Ideally, contraceptive plans should be initiated during the antepartum period. Many adult women choose to return to their preconception method after delivery; however, most pregnant adolescents conceive while not using contraception, and many have no prior experience with contraception. Others conceived after contraceptive failure, often due to incorrect method use. Healthcare providers play an important role in educating teens about all methods of contraception and enabling access to more effective, long-acting reversible contraceptives.

Evidence of Effective Strategies

Since the advent of modern contraceptives, the prevalence of unintended pregnancy among women who state a desire to avoid conception has mystified professionals. It is evident that more is needed than just availability of safe contraceptive methods. A multitude of interventions have been attempted to prevent second births at a young age among adolescent mothers. These include home-visiting programs, which seem to improve teens' attitudes about parenting without decreasing the repeat pregnancy rate [45]; "Dollar-a-day" programs which pay young women to remain nonpregnant which have been unsuccessful [46]; and cell phone-based counseling interventions [47]. Other social interventions such as frequent clinic visits and contact with supportive healthcare providers have also not demonstrated a benefit of delaying repeat pregnancy among adolescent mothers. Because school failure and dropout have been associated with repeat adolescent pregnancy, programs to keep adolescents in school or help them return to school have been attempted [8, 46]. Unfortunately, these too have not demonstrated a reduction in repeat teen pregnancy. This may be because logistical barriers and lack of contraceptive information are not at the root of repeat adolescent childbearing. Rather, the motivation to remain nonpregnant in young women who do not see pregnancy as interfering with future goals is insufficient to support long-term contraceptive use [14]. Interestingly, programs that have shown success in reducing rapid-repeat teen pregnancy rely on motivation-independent methods, such as IUDs and subdermal implants [8, 36, 48].

The immediate postpartum period is an ideal time to initiate long-acting reversible contraceptives. IUDs can be safely placed immediately postpartum after a vaginal or cesarean delivery [49]. However, one study found that in postpartum adolescents, the subdermal implant was more likely to be received prior to resumption of intercourse than the IUD [48]. Another study found that placing subdermal implants prior to hospital discharge in adolescent mothers resulted in a tenfold decrease in the 2-year repeat pregnancy rate, from 41 to 4.2 % [50].

SUMMARY

Young mothers face a multitude of challenges, spanning changes in body image, sexuality, food and housing stability, and future-oriented goals. Repeat adolescent pregnancy is extremely common, ranging from 30 to 44 % within 2 years in most studies, and results in a greater likelihood of persistent poverty, as well as worse health and social outcomes for the mother and her children.

While most contraceptives are safe for postpartum adolescents, even those who are breastfeeding, research over the last 15 years has consistently shown that little besides motivation-independent, reversible contraception delays rapid-repeat teen pregnancy, with the best outcomes reported for the earliest initiation.

REFERENCES

1. Stevens-Simon C, Kelly L, Singer D. Absence of negative attitudes toward childbearing among pregnant teenagers. A risk factor for a rapid repeat pregnancy? Arch Pediatr Adolesc Med. 1996;150(10): 1037–43.
2. Schelar E, Franzetta K, Manlove J. Repeat teen childbearing: differences across states and by race and ethnicity. Washington, D.C.: Child Trends; 2007. Contract No.: 2007–23.
3. Klerman LV, Baker BA, Howard G. Second births among teenage mothers: program results and statistical methods. J Adolesc Health. 2003;32(6):452–5.
4. Klerman LV. The intendedness of pregnancy: a concept in transition. Matern Child Health J. 2000;4(3):155–62.
5. Meade CS, Ickovics JR. Systematic review of sexual risk among pregnant and mothering teens in the USA: pregnancy as an opportunity for integrated prevention of STD and repeat pregnancy. Soc Sci Med. 2005;60(4):661–78.
6. Mott FL. The pace of repeated childbearing among young American mothers. Fam Plann Perspect. 1986;18(1):5–12.
7. Stevens-Simon C, Parsons J, Montgomery C. What is the relationship between postpartum withdrawal from school and repeat pregnancy among adolescent mothers? J Adolesc Health Care. 1986; 7(3):191–4.
8. Stevens-Simon C, Kelly L, Kulick R. A village would be nice but… it takes a long-acting contraceptive to prevent repeat adolescent pregnancies. Am J Prev Med. 2001;21(1):60–5.
9. Reubinoff BE, Grubstein A, Meirow D, Berry E, Schenker JG, Brzezinski A. Effects of low-dose estrogen oral contraceptives on weight, body composition, and fat distribution in young women. Fertil Steril. 1995;63(3):516–21.
10. Lloyd T, Lin HM, Matthews AE, Bentley CM, Legro RS. Oral contraceptive use by teenage women does not affect body composition. Obstet Gynecol. 2002;100(2):235–9.
11. Harel Z, Biro FM, Kollar LM, Rauh JL. Adolescents' reasons for and experience after discontinuation of the long-acting contraceptives Depo-Provera and Norplant. J Adolesc Health. 1996;19(2): 118–23.
12. O'Dell CM, Forke CM, Polaneczky MM, Sondheimer SJ, Slap GB. Depot medroxyprogesterone acetate or oral contraception in postpartum adolescents. Obstet Gynecol. 1998;91(4):609–14.
13. Bonny AE, Ziegler J, Harvey R, Debanne SM, Secic M, Cromer BA. Weight gain in obese and nonobese adolescent girls initiating

depot medroxyprogesterone, oral contraceptive pills, or no hormonal contraceptive method. Arch Pediatr Adolesc Med. 2006; 160(1):40–5.

14. Sheeder J, Tocce K, Stevens-Simon C. Reasons for ineffective contraceptive use antedating adolescent pregnancies part 1: an indicator of gaps in family planning services. Matern Child Health J. 2009;13(3):295–305.

15. Schmidt RM, Wiemann CM, Rickert VI, Smith EO. Moderate to severe depressive symptoms among adolescent mothers followed four years postpartum. J Adolesc Health. 2006;38(6):712–8.

16. Sheeder J, Kabir K, Stafford B. Screening for postpartum depression at well-child visits: is once enough during the first 6 months of life? Pediatrics. 2009;123(6):e982–8.

17. Rigsby DC, Macones GA, Driscoll DA. Risk factors for rapid repeat pregnancy among adolescent mothers: a review of the literature. J Pediatr Adolesc Gynecol. 1998;11(3):115–26.

18. Centers for Disease Control and Prevention (CDC). U.S. Medical Eligibility Criteria for Contraceptive Use, 2010. MMWR Recomm Rep. 2010;59(RR–4):1–86.

19. American College of Obstetricians and Gynecologists. ACOG Committee Opinion No. 361. Breastfeeding: maternal and infant aspects. Obstet Gynecol. 2007;109(2 Pt 1):479–80.

20. Centers for Disease Control and Prevention (CDC). Breastfeeding trends and updated national health objectives for exclusive breastfeeding–United States, birth years 2000–2004. MMWR Morb Mortal Wkly Rep. 2007;56(30):760–3.

21. Truitt ST, Fraser AB, Grimes DA, Gallo MF, Schulz KF. Hormonal contraception during lactation. Systematic review of randomized controlled trials. Contraception. 2003;68(4):233–8.

22. Stanwood NL, Garrett JM, Konrad TR. Obstetrician-gynecologists and the intrauterine device: a survey of attitudes and practice. Obstet Gynecol. 2002;99(2):275–80.

23. Harper CC, Blum M, de Bocanegra HT, Darney PD, Speidel JJ, Policar M, et al. Challenges in translating evidence to practice: the provision of intrauterine contraception. Obstet Gynecol. 2008; 111(6):1359–69.

24. Committee on Adolescent Health Care Long-Acting Reversible Contraception Working Group, The American College of Obstetricians and Gynecologists. Committee opinion no. 539: adolescents and long-acting reversible contraception: implants and intrauterine devices. Obstet Gynecol. 2012;120(4):983–8.

25. LAM effective but inconvenient for women in the U.S. Contracept Technol Update. 1993;14(3):48–50.

26. Geerling JH. Natural family planning. Am Fam Physician. 1995; 52(6):1749–56, 59–60.

27. Guida M, Tommaselli GA, Pellicano M, Palomba S, Nappi C. An overview on the effectiveness of natural family planning. Gynecol Endocrinol. 1997;11(3):203–19.

28. Labbok MH, Perez A, Valdes V, Sevilla F, Wade K, Laukaran VH, et al. The lactational amenorrhea method (LAM): a postpartum introductory family planning method with policy and program implications. Adv Contracept. 1994;10(2):93–109.

29. Feldman-Winter L, Shaikh U. Optimizing breastfeeding promotion and support in adolescent mothers. J Hum Lact. 2007;23(4): 362–7.

30. Spear HJ. Breastfeeding behaviors and experiences of adolescent mothers. MCN Am J Matern Child Nurs. 2006;31(2):106–13.

31. Centers for Disease Control and Prevention. Update to CDC's U.S. Medical Eligibility Criteria for Contraceptive Use, 2010: revised recommendations for the use of contraceptive methods during the postpartum period. MMWR Morb Mortal Wkly Rep. 2011;60(26): 878–83.

32. Kapp N, Curtis K, Nanda K. Progestogen-only contraceptive use among breastfeeding women: a systematic review. Contraception. 2010;82(1):17–37.

33. Sivin I, Diaz S, Croxatto HB, Miranda P, Shaaban M, Sayed EH, et al. Contraceptives for lactating women: a comparative trial of a progesterone-releasing vaginal ring and the copper T 380A IUD. Contraception. 1997;55(4):225–32.

34. Medical eligibility criteria for contraceptive use. 4th ed. Geneva: World Health Organization; 2010. http://www.who.int/reproductive-health/publications/mec/mec.pdf. Accessed 25 Oct 2010.

35. American College of Obstetricians and Gynecologists. ACOG Practice Bulletin No. 121. Long-acting reversible contraception: Implants and Intrauterine devices. Obstet Gynecol. 2011;118: 184–96.

36. Lewis LN, Doherty DA, Hickey M, Skinner SR. Implanon as a con-traceptive choice for teenage mothers: a comparison of contracep-tive choices, acceptability and repeat pregnancy. Contraception. 2010;81(5):421–6.

37. Polaneczky M, Slap G, Forke C, Rappaport A, Sondheimer S. The use of levonorgestrel implants (Norplant) for contraception in ado-lescent mothers. N Engl J Med. 1994;331(18):1201–6.

38. Stevens-Simon C, Kelly L. Correlates and consequences of early removal of levonorgestrel implants among teenaged mothers. Arch Pediatr Adolesc Med. 1998;152(9):893–8.

39. Gurtcheff SE, Turok DK, Stoddard G, Murphy PA, Gibson M, Jones KP. Lactogenesis after early postpartum use of the contraceptive implant: a randomized controlled trial. Obstet Gynecol. 2011; 117(5):1114–21. Epub 2011/04/22.

40. Rodriguez MI, Kaunitz AM. An evidence-based approach to post-partum use of depot medroxyprogesterone acetate in breastfeeding women. Contraception. 2009;80(1):4–6.

41. Taneepanichskul S, Reinprayoon D, Thaithumyanon P, Praisuwanna P, Tosukhowong P, Dieben T. Effects of the etonogestrel-releasing implant Implanon and a nonmedicated intrauterine device on the growth of breast-fed infants. Contraception. 2006;73(4):368–71.

42. American College of Obstetricians and Gynecologists. ACOG Committee Opinion No. 392, December 2007. Intrauterine device and adolescents. Obstet Gynecol. 2007;110(6):1493–5.
43. Rodrigues da Cunha AC, Dorea JG, Cantuaria AA. Intrauterine device and maternal copper metabolism during lactation. Contraception. 2001;63(1):37–9.
44. Shaamash AH, Sayed GH, Hussien MM, Shaaban MM. A comparative study of the levonorgestrel-releasing intrauterine system Mirena versus the Copper T380A intrauterine device during lactation: breast-feeding performance, infant growth and infant development. Contraception. 2005;72(5):346–51.
45. Barnet B, Liu J, DeVoe M, Alperovitz-Bichell K, Duggan AK. Home visiting for adolescent mothers: effects on parenting, maternal life course, and primary care linkage. Ann Fam Med. 2007;5(3): 224–32.
46. Stevens-Simon C, Dolgan JI, Kelly L, Singer D. The effect of monetary incentives and peer support groups on repeat adolescent pregnancies. A randomized trial of the Dollar-a-Day Program. JAMA. 1997;277(12):977–82.
47. Katz KS, Rodan M, Milligan R, Tan S, Courtney L, Gantz M, et al. Efficacy of a randomized cell phone-based counseling intervention in postponing subsequent pregnancy among teen mothers. Matern Child Health J. 2011;15 Suppl 1:S42–53. Epub 2011/08/03.
48. Tocce K, Sheeder J, Python J, Teal SB. Long acting reversible contraception in postpartum adolescents: early initiation of etonogestrel implant is superior to IUDs in the outpatient setting. J Pediatr Adolesc Gynecol. 2012;25(1):59–63.
49. Kapp N, Curtis KM. Intrauterine device insertion during the postpartum period: a systematic review. Contraception. 2009;80(4): 327–36.
50. Tocce K, Sheeder J, Teal S. Offering adolescents immediate postpartum etonogestrel implant: 2-year continuation and repeat pregnancy rates. Contraception. 2012;86(3):295.

Chapter 12
Sexuality Education

Melissa Kottke

Sexuality is how people experience and express themselves as sexual beings. Sexuality is far more than sexual intercourse and its outcomes. It is a fundamental part of being human that has impact on broad aspects of human life from physical, social, and psychological to economic, spiritual, cultural, and political. Thus, a parallel definition of sexuality education includes that which goes beyond physical sexual behaviors and outcomes. One suggestion set as a goal for sexuality education is "an age-appropriate, culturally relevant approach to teaching about sex and relationships by providing scientifically accurate, realistic, non-judgmental information. Sexuality education provides opportunities to explore one's own values and attitudes and to build decision-making, communication, and risk reduction skills about many aspects of sexuality" [1]. This chapter will review the rationale for sexuality education and current opinions on best practices for sexuality education and provide pragmatic suggestions for clinicians.

RATIONALE FOR SEXUALITY EDUCATION
Human adolescence is marked by sexual maturation and growth. While the transformation to a sexual being is human, involuntary, and inevitable, the transformation to a *healthy* sexual being is not. Education about this evolving sexuality is the cornerstone of prevention in the field of adolescent sexual and reproductive health

M. Kottke, M.D., M.P.H. (✉)
Department of Gynecology and Obstetrics, Emory University,
1256 Briarcliff Road, Atlanta, GA 30306, USA
e-mail: mkottke@emory.edu

A. Whitaker and M. Gilliam (eds.), *Contraception for Adolescent and Young Adult Women*, DOI 10.1007/978-1-4614-6579-9_12,
© Springer Science+Business Media New York 2014

(ASRH), and a lack of education on sexuality leaves one vulnerable to a range of issues. Most commonly, the high rates of physical sexual health outcomes are highlighted as evidence for the need for sexuality education. For example:

- The USA has one of the highest teen pregnancy rates in the developed world [2].
- Every year three quarters of a million teens get pregnant in the USA [3].
- Eighty percent of these pregnancies are unintended [4].
- Young people account for nearly half of all sexually transmitted infections (STDs) reported in the USA each year and now account for the largest age group of those diagnosed with HIV each year [5, 6].

But what is not as frequently discussed are the negative outcomes associated with a broader context of sexuality.

- Nearly 90 % of lesbian, gay, bisexual, and transgendered (LGBT) students report being harassed during the previous year [7].
- Nationally, 10 % of high school students indicate that they were hit, slapped, or hurt on purpose by a dating partner [8].
- Nearly one in three sexually active adolescent girls in 9th–12th grade (31.5 %) report ever experiencing physical or sexual violence from dating partners [9].
- According to the National Survey for Family Growth, among those who had had sexual intercourse before the age of 20, 59 % of females and 38 % of males reported that they did not want to have sex at that time or had mixed feelings about it [10].

As a precursor to these outcomes, data looking into adolescent's knowledge of sexual and reproductive health also indicate important gaps. A recent report from the Pregnancy Risk Assessment Monitoring System asked teen mothers 15–19 years old who did not use contraception at the time of unintended pregnancy why they did not use contraception. Nearly one third (31 %) indicated they did not think they could get pregnant at the time. Nearly one quarter (23 %) indicated their partner did not want them to use contraception, 22 % did not mind if they get pregnant, 13 % had difficulty getting contraception, 9 % were fearful of contraceptive side effects, and 8 % thought they were infertile [11]. According to the Fog Zone, published by the National Campaign to Prevent Teen and Unintended Pregnancy, these gaps in knowledge and behavior extend to the young adult years, as well. Among those 18–29 who were surveyed, 30 % say they know *little or nothing* about condoms, 63 % say they know *little or nothing* about birth control pills, and 56 % say they have *not heard* of the birth control implant. Furthermore, much like the parenting teens in the PRAMS studied above, misinformation about pregnancy and contraception was common. Forty percent of the young adults (those who were relying on withdrawal or natural family planning) did not know when during the menstrual cycle a woman is most fertile. Over one quarter (27 %) of unmarried young women believe that it is *extremely or quite likely* that using birth control pills or other hormonal methods of contraception for a long period of time will lead to a serious health problem like cancer. Over one third (36 %) say it is likely that the pill will cause them to gain weight, and 40 % say it will likely cause *severe* mood swings *and* that these concerns reduce the likelihood of their using the pill. Nearly one in five (19 %) young adult women thought it was quite or extremely likely she was infertile. And even among those who say it is important to them to avoid pregnancy right now, 20 % of women and 43 % of men say they would be at least a little pleased if they found out today that they or their partner were pregnant [12].

The PRAMS study and the Fog Zone highlight the need for improved education on key topics: how/when pregnancy occurs, how to access contraception, contraceptive safety, and fertility realities. Furthermore, they highlight the need to approach sexuality education from beyond only the physical sexual health outcomes. With sexuality education, young people should also explore relationships and communication within them as well as pregnancy and parenting motivations. These studies also suggest that the current approach to sexuality education may have important deficits and that sexuality education should be presented as an iterative process, with ongoing application and reassessment as one grows, and acknowledgment that sex, relationships, and fertility are powerful components of our lives.

There is broad support for sexuality education. In 2004, National Public Radio (NPR), the Kaiser Family Foundation, and the Kennedy School of Government released a poll that indicated that only 7 % of Americans thought that sexuality education should not be taught in schools. The study found that there was great variation in opinions about what kind of sexuality education should be taught, with 15 % preferring abstinence only, 36 % supporting education that focuses on responsible decisions about sex, and 46 % supporting "abstinence-plus" [13]. From a public health perspective, reproductive and sexual health is one of the twelve Leading Health Indicators for Healthy People 2020. Indeed, there are many objectives in these national health goals that are linked to sexuality education for young people, one explicitly, including [14]:

- Family planning (FP)-8: Reduce pregnancy rates among adolescent females.
- FP-9: Increase the proportion of adolescents aged 17 years and under who have never had sexual intercourse.
- FP-10: Increase the proportion of sexually active persons aged 15–19 years who use condoms to both effectively prevent pregnancy and provide barrier protection against disease.
- FP-11: Increase the proportion of sexually active persons aged 15–19 years who use condoms and hormonal or intrauterine contraception to both effectively prevent.
- FP-12 Increase the proportion of adolescents who received formal instruction on reproductive health topics before they were 18 years old.
- FP-13 Increase the proportion of adolescents who talked to a parent or guardian about reproductive health topics before they were 18 years old.
- STD-1: Reduce the proportion of adolescents and young adults with Chlamydia trachomatis infections.
- STD-6: Reduce gonorrhea rates.
- HIV-1: Reduce the number of new HIV diagnoses among adolescents and adults.

Recent efforts from the Centers for Disease Control and Prevention have also expanded the public health framework of sexual health to be more broadly inclusive of aspects beyond physical and sexual health. The external consultation identified six objectives for a new sexual health framework [15].

- Increase healthy, responsible, and respectful sexual behaviors and attitudes.
- Increase the awareness and ability to make healthy and responsible choices, free of coercion.
- Promote healthy sexual functioning and relationships, including ensuring that individuals have control over, and decide freely on, matters related to their own sexual relations and health.
- Optimize and educate about reproductive health.
- Increase access to effective preventive, screening, treatment, and support services that promote sexual health.
- Decrease adverse individual and public health outcomes including HIV/STDs, viral hepatitis, unintended pregnancies, and sexual violence.

Even with general acceptance and acknowledgment of sexual health risks and goals, there is disagreement as to how best to accomplish these goals within sexuality education. A common concern raised about sexuality education is that by teaching young people about sex and sexuality, risky behaviors will be encouraged or hastened. Reviews of sexuality programs from the USA and internationally indicate that this fear is not the case. UNESCO and Kirby reviewed 87 sex and STD/HIV education curricula that reported outcomes on sexual behaviors (initiation of sex, frequency of sex, number of sex partners, use of condoms, use of contraception, and sexual risk taking). The findings reveal an increase in protective behaviors or no significant difference for each of the behaviors in greater than 93 % of studies [1, 16].

Other recent empirical data also support the practice of sexuality education for young people. A recent study from the Guttmacher Institute used data from the NSFG including 4,691 male and female individuals aged 15–24. They found that receipt of sex education, regardless of type (only abstinence, abstinence and birth control, or neither), was associated with delays in first sex for both genders, as compared to receiving no sex education. Those who received instruction about abstinence and birth control were significantly more likely at first sex to use any contraception, more likely to use a condom, and less likely to have an age-discrepant partner. Receipt of only abstinence education was not statistically distinguishable in most models from receipt of either both or neither topics. Among female subjects, condom use at first sex was significantly more likely among those receiving instruction in both topics as compared with only abstinence education [17]. This finding is particularly salient because contraception use at first sex is an important correlate for teen pregnancy. Previous reports from the NSFG have found that the probability of pregnancy between ages 15 and 19 was nearly double for those who did not use a contraceptive method at first sex compared to those who did [10].

BEST PRACTICES

Though informal sexuality education (via media, online, peer environments, etc.) is powerful, much of the conversation around sexuality education in the USA is focused on formal avenues for sexuality education (schools and other settings for curricula delivery). A systematic review by the Community Preventive Services Task Force [18] reviewed 89 adolescent sexual and reproductive health interventions (66 that were comprehensive risk reduction, 23 that were abstinence only) that took place in a diversity of settings (in schools and in community-based programs).

Their synthesis found sufficient evidence to recommend group-based comprehensive risk reduction delivered to adolescents to promote behaviors that prevent or reduce the risk of pregnancy, HIV, and other STIDs. The Task Force identified that group-based comprehensive risk reduction was successful at reducing a number of self-reported risk behaviors (engagement in any sexual activity, frequency of sexual activity, number of sex partners, and frequency of unprotected sexual activity, increasing the self-reported use of protection against pregnancy and STDs and reducing the incidence of self-reported or clinically documented STDs). They found the results from group-based abstinence-only education to be inconclusive due to inconsistent effects on the studied outcomes [19].

The Future of Sex Education (FoSE) project was started in 2007 focused solely on the in-school setting for sexuality education. It brought together key organizations that were already central in the sex education dialogue in the USA; the purpose was "to create a national dialogue about the future of sex education and to promote the institutionalization of comprehensive sexuality education in public schools." The three primary organizations that comprised FoSE were Advocates for Youth, Answer, and SEICUS (Sexuality Information and Education Council of the United States). In 2011, FoSE released the National Sexuality Education Standards. This document puts forth the minimum core content and skills responsive to the needs of students and in service to their overall academic achievement and sexual health. The standards identify seven topic areas (anatomy and physiology, puberty and adolescent development, identity, pregnancy and reproduction, sexually transmitted diseases and HIV, healthy relationships, and personal safety). The National Sexuality Education Standards organized its recommendations with the National Health Education Standards, which has eight categories of its own (core content, analyze influencers, access information, interpersonal communication, decision-making, goal setting, self-management, and advocacy). The National Sexuality Education Standards offer detailed performance indicators of what students should know or be able to do at the end of grades 2, 5, 8, and 12. The standards set expectations of each of the seven topics in each of the eight categories for each of the age levels. For example, under anatomy and physiology and core content, by the end of 2nd grade a student should be able to "explain that all living things reproduce," under healthy relationships and interpersonal communication by the end of 8th grade, they should be able to "demonstrate the communication skills that foster healthy relationships," and under personal safety and analyzing influences, by the end of 12th grade, they should be able to "describe potential impacts of power differences (e.g., age, status or position) within sexual relationships" [20]. In addition to the formalizing the standards, FoSE also offers professional development opportunities for advocates and educators to work with legislators and decision makers at the national, state, and local levels, as well as the general public, to make decisions that support adolescent reproductive and sexual health.

As it is a universal concern, efforts to guide the content of sexuality education are not limited to the USA. The International Technical Guidelines on Sexuality Education were published by a multidisciplinary, multinational collaborative by UNESCO in 2009. Similar to FoSE, this guidance suggests sexuality education should be approached via six key topics (relationships; values, attitudes, and skills; culture, society, and human rights; human development; sexual behavior; sexual and reproductive health) with different components delivered between the ages of 5 and 18 when developmentally appropriate. This guidance identified key ingredients shared by effective sexuality education programs in that they:

- Reduce misinformation.
- Increase correct knowledge.
- Clarify and strengthen positive values and attitudes.
- Increase skills to make informed decisions and act upon them.
- Improve perceptions about peer groups and social norms.
- Increase communication with parents or other trusted adults.

Both FoSE and the International Technical Guidelines on Sexuality Education reflect the increasing recognition that a singular focus on physical sexual health risk reduction (i.e., how to avoid pregnancy and/or STIs) is insufficient to promote healthy sexuality. Sexuality has myriad influencers. These influencing factors include the broader contextual influences of gender, human rights and culture, as well as individual values, attitudes, and experiences. Emerging approaches to sexuality education engage with this range of influences. For example, DiClemente and Wingood have developed several curricula to increase condom use and decrease STIs/HIV. Their programs are interactive and address issues of gender and ethnic pride, self-esteem, and self-awareness [21–23]. Amy Schalet has explored the importance of culture and context in her studies of the different approaches to adolescent sexuality in the USA and in the Netherlands. She sheds light upon the "dramatization" of adolescent sexuality as something to be feared and forbidden that is seen in the USA and compares that to the acceptance of sexuality, the support of loving relationships, and the setting of clear expectations that is more common in the Netherlands [24]. She proposes a shift in the paradigm of adolescent sexual health using the *ABC and D* framework. With this acronym she suggests that the following components are essential for youth to develop into healthy sexual beings: sexual *autonomy*, *building* good romantic relationships, *connectedness* with a parent or other caregiver(s), and recognizing *diversities* in stages of development and removing *disparities* in access to vital socioeconomic resources. With this approach, young people are provided necessary knowledge and access but are also encouraged to form their own visions and expectations with regard to sexuality [25]. Since 1999, Scenarios USA has been partnering with young people to broaden what sexuality education can be. Using films that explore the realities of youth, sexuality, and its influences, Scenarios USA offers the "REAL DEAL" to young people. These "REAL DEAL" films are written by teens and for teens. They present complex situations and characters that resonate with teens and may help young people see the impact of (and begin to analyze) these broader influences of race, gender, and class on them as individuals, their approach to sexual expression, and their decision-making [26]. As a final example, in 2011 the Population Council introduced an evidence-based curriculum called *It's All One*. One of the most comprehensive curricula on sexuality education, this curriculum is intended for global audiences and has its foundation in the universal principles of gender equality and human rights. Not only is this curriculum comprehensive (unit topics include the following: sexual health and well-being require human rights, gender, sexuality, interpersonal relationships, communication and decision-making skills, the body, puberty and reproduction, sexual and reproductive health (including HIV prevention and contraception), and advocating for sexual health, rights, and gender equality), it also works to integrate these topics recognizing that these different influences are interconnected and this interconnectedness impacts sexual health. It acknowledges that the needs for sexuality education are not predetermined and may vary over time and by age, geography, culture, and political and religious context and, thus, encourages adaptations to development level and local milieu. This work redefines what sexuality education can be and is inspiring in scope and aim, "...the ultimate goal of *It's All One Curriculum* is to develop the capacity of young people to enjoy— and advocate for their rights to—dignity, equality, and responsible, satisfying, and healthy sexual lives" [27].

SUGGESTIONS FOR CLINICIANS

While the above guidelines suggest ingredients of successful formal sexuality education programming, it is clear that clinicians can facilitate much in the clinical setting. Young people trust their clinicians when it comes to sexual and reproductive health questions, and nearly half report their physician as a key informant for learning about birth control and STD protection [28, 29]. Clinicians have unique opportunities to provide meaningful sexuality education and/or augment previous lessons learned. Indeed, each clinical encounter lends an opportunity to do so, and this is likely true throughout the lifespan and across genders. There is little guidance, but promising techniques may include:

- Set the stage for education about sexuality by bringing it up at regular intervals. The adolescent's context changes rapidly and clinicians should discuss sexuality frequently. Not only does frequent discussion demonstrate that sexuality is an important part of health and health care, but it also may open the door for the patient to ask questions or bring up concerns in future visits. Use of the HEEADSSS model (Home, Education, Eating, Activities, Drugs, Sexuality, Suicide/Depression, Safety) during the interview of the adolescent ensures that sexuality is discussed consistently
- Young people are more likely to present their truths and take away educational pearls from a supportive and nonjudgmental interaction. It may be useful to engage in self-reflection about your thoughts on adolescent sexuality, your comfort in talking concretely about sex with teens, and how your language (verbal and nonverbal) is interpreted by others. Practice gender-neutral conversations as your patient may be seeking a safe space to discuss sexual identity and orientation.
- Take a thorough sexual history keeping in mind the concrete nature of the developing adolescent mind. Asking open-ended questions is enlightening and may provide valuable opportunities to correct misinformation as well as insights into unrealized risks. There are myriad myths surrounding sexuality; asking open-ended questions may uncover one. As an example from one of my patients, the question, "tell me about how your partner uses a condom," revealed that the condom was placed after the initiation of intercourse during a pause just before ejaculation. Asking this patient "do you and your partner use condoms?" would have gotten a "yes" response, and we both would have been satisfied, but it would have been a missed opportunity. This answer prompted education about the optimal

use of condoms, as well as skill building on how to place a condom on a partner (and when it should be on), and how to communicate about its use.

- Ask about your patient's relationships. Relationships are important and partners are influential in decision-making around sexual and reproductive health issues. What does the relationship offer? Are there signs of abuse? (physical, sexual, emotional, etc.)

- Seek ways to provide education in an experiential format, when possible. Have them practice. "Describe for me how you will use the patch." Challenge them with scenarios that may arise, "and what if it falls off?" Role play. "How are you going to discuss condom use with your partner? You play you, I'll be your partner...."

- Using motivational interviewing techniques may be useful in framing the conversation. Identifying the patient's goals, clarifying the behaviors, confirming understanding of the outcomes associated with behaviors, and helping the young person draw linkages between behaviors, outcomes, and goals may be a powerful tool not only in suggesting behavior change but also in reaffirming positive decisions made.

- Arrange for frequent follow-up for young patients. Relationships and situations change rapidly. Clinicians can help a young person navigate these changes in a healthy way. Frequent follow-up can allow for incremental problem solving and avoid overwhelming a young person with everything they ever needed to know about sexuality during one clinical visit.

- Make your clinical site a place for obtaining sexuality education information. Techniques include using pamphlets, posters, waiting room videos, etc. Many resources can be age, gender, and culturally specific to fit with your clinical population. See Table 12.1.

- Become knowledgeable about your state's laws regarding sexuality education (available at the Guttmacher Institute, see Table 12.1) as well as local school- and community-based efforts. This awareness will help you understand what your patients may know, where gaps may be, and where in the community you can refer if the need arises.

- Seek ways to provide sexuality education in formal settings (schools, community, and faith-based organizations) if this topic is interesting to you; your medical insights are valuable and respected.

TABLE 12.1 Sexuality education resources.

Sexuality education resources	
Advocates for Youth	http://www.advocatesforyouth.org/
Answer	http://answer.rutgers.edu/page/lesson_plans/
Future of Sex Education Initiative	http://www.futureofsexed.org/index.html
It's All One	http://www.itsallone.org/
Guttmacher Institute (state-specific sex education requirements)	http://www.guttmacher.org/statecenter/ spibs/spib_SE.pdf
Resource Center for Adolescent Pregnancy Prevention	http://recapp.etr.org/recapp/
Scenarios, USA	https://www.scenariosusa.org/
The Sex Ed Library by SIECUS	http://www.sexedlibrary.org/

CONCLUSION

Sexuality education is critical for health and wellness on an individual and population level. Outcome and knowledge evidence suggests that substantial gaps remain regarding sexuality education. Best practices in sexuality education vary; however, key ingredients have surfaced including the need for sexuality education beyond isolated physical sexual health, the need for accurate information, and the need for education to be delivered over time when developmentally appropriate. Clinicians can play a vital role in introducing and/or reinforcing sexuality education for their patients during the clinical encounter.

REFERENCES

1. UNESCO, International Technical Guidance on Sexuality Education, Dec 2009. http://www.ibe.unesco.org/fileadmin/user_upload/HIV_and_AIDS/documents/UNESCO_Guidelines_Sexuality_Education.pdf
2. McKay A, Barrett M. Trends in teen pregnancy rates from 1996–2006: a comparison of Canada, Sweden, USA and England/Wales. Can J Hum Sex. 2010;19(1–2):43–52.
3. Kost K, Henshaw S, Carlin L. U.S. teenage pregnancies, births and abortions: national and state trends and trends by race and ethnicity. New York, NY: Guttmacher Institute; 2010. http://www.guttmacher.org/pubs/USTPtrends.pdf.

4. Finer LB, Zolna MR. Unintended pregnancy in the United States: incidence and disparities, 2006. Contraception. 2011;84(5):478–85. doi:10.1016/j.contraception.2011.07.013.

5. Centers for Disease Control and Prevention. HIV Surveillance Report, 2009;21. http://www.cdc.gov/hiv/surveillance/resources/reports/2009report/pdf/cover.pdf. Diagnoses of HIV infection by age. http://www.cdc.gov/hiv/topics/surveillance/basic.htm#hivaidsage

6. Centers for Disease Control and Prevention. STD Surveillance 2010. http://www.cdc.gov/std/stats10/default.htm

7. Kosciw JG, et al. The 2009 National School Climate Survey: the experiences of lesbian, gay, bisexual and transgender youth in our nation's schools. New York: GLSEN; 2010.

8. Centers for Disease Control and Prevention. Youth risk behavioral surveillance—United States, 2009. Morb Mortal Wkly Rep. 2010; 59(S1–5):1–148.

9. Decker M, Silverman J, Raj A. Dating violence and sexually transmitted disease/HIV testing and diagnosis among adolescent females. Pediatrics. 2005;116:272–6.

10. Martinez G, Copen CE, Abma JC. Teenagers in the United States: Sexual activity, contraceptive use, and childbearing, 2006–2010 National Survey of Family Growth. Vital Health Stat 23. 2011; 31:1–35.

11. Centers for Disease Control and Prevention. Prepregnancy contraceptive Use among teens with unintended pregnancies resulting in live births—Pregnancy Risk Assessment Monitoring System (PRAMS), 2004–2008. MMWR Morb Mortal Wkly Rep. 2012;61:25–9.

12. Kaye K, Suellentrop K, Sloup C. The fog zone: how misperceptions, magical thinking, and ambivalence put young adults at risk for unplanned pregnancy. Washington, DC: The National Campaign to Prevent Teen and Unplanned Pregnancy; 2009.

13. NPR, Kaiser Family Foundation, Kennedy School of Government. Sex education in America: general public/parents survey. 2004.

14. U.S. Department of Health and Human Services. Office of Disease Prevention and Health Promotion. Healthy People 2020. Washington, DC. http://www.healthypeople.gov/2020/LHI/reproductiveHealth.aspx

15. Centers for Disease Control and Prevention. A public health approach for advancing sexual health in the United States: rationale and options for implementation, meeting report of an external consultation. Atlanta, GA: Centers for Disease Control and Prevention; 2010.

16. Kirby D. Emerging Answers 2007: research findings on programs to reduce teen pregnancy and sexually transmitted diseases. Washington, DC: National Campaign to Prevent Teen and Unplanned Pregnancy; 2007.

17. Lindberg LD, Maddow-Zimet I. Consequences of sex education on teen and young adult sexual behaviors and outcomes. J Adolesc Health. 2012;51(4):332–8. http://dx.doi.org/10.1016/j.jadohealth.2011.12.028.

18. Community Preventive Task Force. Recommendations for group-based behavioral interventions to prevent adolescent pregnancy, human immunodeficiency virus, and other sexually transmitted infections: comprehensive risk reduction and abstinence education. Am J Prev Med. 2012;42(3):304–7.
19. Chin H, Sipe T, Community Preventive Services Task Force, et al. The effectiveness of group-based comprehensive risk-reduction and abstinence education interventions to prevent or reduce the risk of adolescent pregnancy, human immunodeficiency virus, and sexually transmitted infections two systematic reviews for the guide to community preventive services. Am J Prev Med. 2012;42(3):272–94.
20. Future of Sex Education Initiative. (2012). National Sexuality Education Standards: core content and skills, K-12 [a special publication of the Journal of School Health]. http://www.futureofsex-education.org/documents/josh-fose-standards-web.pdf
21. DiClemente RJ, Wingood GM. A randomized controlled trial of an HIV sexual risk-reduction intervention for young African-American women. JAMA. 1995;274(16):1271–6.
22. DiClemente RJ, Wingood GM, Harrington KF, Lang DL, Davies SL, Hook 3rd EW, Oh MK, Crosby RA, Hertzberg VS, Gordon AB, Hardin JW, Parker S, Robillard A. Efficacy of an HIV prevention intervention for African American adolescent girls: a randomized controlled trial. JAMA. 2004;292(2):171–9.
23. DiClemente RJ, Wingood GM, Rose ES, Sales JM, Lang DL, Caliendo AM, Hardin JW, Crosby RA. Efficacy of sexually transmitted disease/human immunodeficiency virus sexual risk-reduction intervention for African American adolescent females seeking sexual health services. Arch Pediatr Adolesc Med. 2009; 163(12):1112–21.
24. Schalet AT. Beyond abstinence and risk: a new paradigm for adolescent sexual health. Womens Health Issues. 2011;21(3S):S5–7.
25. Schalet AT. Not under my roof: parents, teens and the culture of sex. Chicago: University of Chicago Press; 2011.
26. Scenarios USA. http://www.scenariosusa.org/.
27. Population Council. It's All One Curriculum. 2011. www.itsallone.org
28. Kaiser Family Foundation, Seventeen Magazine. Sex smarts: birth control and protection. Menlo Park, CA: Kaiser Family Foundation; 2004.
29. Strasburger VC. Adolescents, sex and the media: Ooooo, baby, baby. A Q&A. Adolesc Med Clin. 2005;16:269–88.

Chapter 13
Legal and Policy Issues
in Adolescent Contraceptive Care

Lee Hasselbacher

This chapter addresses legal and policy issues that may arise in the context of providing contraceptive care and counseling to adolescents, specifically adolescents who are minors. In particular, the chapter will focus on how issues such as consent and confidentiality can influence the provision of contraceptive care to minors. The broad legal framework for understanding consent and confidentiality in adolescent health care is shaped by federal and state constitutions and statutes, regulations issued by administrative agencies, and cases decided by courts. Given the complex interplay of laws and the resulting state variations in policy, this chapter explores the broader issues regarding provision of contraceptive counseling and services to adolescent.

MINOR CONSENT FOR CONTRACEPTIVE SERVICES

Adolescents who have reached the "age of majority" are able to consent to their own medical care as adults. The age of majority in most states is 18, though in two states (AL, NE) it is 19 and in two other states (MS, PA) it is 21. Minors typically need parental consent to obtain medical care, but there are many exceptions. In emergencies, care may often be provided without the prior consent of a parent, but the health care provider is usually required to inform the parent as soon as possible [1]. Additional federal and

L. Hasselbacher, J.D. (✉)
Section of Family Planning and Contraceptive Research,
Department of Obstetrics and Gynecology, University of Chicago Medicine,
5841 S. Maryland Avenue, MC 2050, Chicago, IL 60637, USA
e-mail: lhasselbacher@uchicago.edu

A. Whitaker and M. Gilliam (eds.), *Contraception for Adolescent and Young Adult Women*, DOI 10.1007/978-1-4614-6579-9_13,
© Springer Science + Business Media New York 2014

state laws have created a number of exceptions to the rule requiring parental consent. These exceptions can grant minors access to a range of reproductive health care services and the ability to obtain contraception on their own. While research has shown that a parent or guardian is often aware when a minor is seeking contraceptive services [2, 3], these laws reflect the understanding that some adolescents may avoid care if parental involvement is a requirement. This section discusses the laws and legal decisions which allow minors to consent for contraceptive services.

State Laws

Most states have one or more laws that grant either all or some minors the ability to consent to contraceptive services independently. These laws, often referred to as "state minor consent laws," come in different forms, and they are usually based on the *status* of the minor or the *services* sought [1, 4].

State consent laws based on *status* authorize certain categories of minors—such as married minors or minors of a particular age—to consent to medical care. These state laws may directly authorize certain minors to consent to care or they may indicate that minors with a certain status can be found emancipated, a process often done through a court proceeding. Traditionally, the criteria for recognizing a minor as emancipated have included marriage, military service, or living apart from parents and being self-supporting. In some cases, a judge may declare a minor fully emancipated; in other cases he or she may be considered emancipated only for certain purposes [1]. At least 37 states have enacted statutes that explicitly authorize an emancipated minor to consent for health care or note that emancipated minors have adult status; in the remaining states, minors who meet traditional criteria for emancipation should also be recognized as able to consent for health care [1].

A number of state laws allow a minor to consent for a particular *service*, such as contraception, testing for sexually transmitted infections, pregnancy related care, or HIV/AIDS care [1, 5]. Many states expressly authorize minors to consent for contraceptive counseling and care; some of these statutes specify "family planning" or "contraceptive" services, while others specify "pregnancy-related care" or services to "prevent pregnancy" [1].

Most minors in most states are able to consent to contraceptive services under state law; only four states have no explicit policy that allows minors to consent to contraceptive services. Twenty-one states and the District of Columbia explicitly allow all minors to consent to contraceptive services; 25 states have laws which permit minors to consent under one or more specific circumstances [1, 4]. These circumstances can include when the minor is married, a parent, is or has been pregnant, if the minor would otherwise face a health hazard, or if the minor meets other requirements such as reaching a minimum age, being a high school graduate, demonstrating maturity, or receiving a referral from specific professionals (e.g., clergy or physician) [1]. A number of states also provide that if a minor is serving in the military or incarcerated, he or she is able to consent to medical care or is considered emancipated. Additional provisions in some states describe a combined set of circumstances under which a minor may consent to medical care—such as a certain age along with evidence of the minor living apart from parents and managing his or her own financial affairs.

Health care professionals have also relied on the "mature minor" doctrine to provide reproductive health care to minors. The "mature minor" doctrine is a legal concept, which has been expressly accepted by courts in several states. Under the doctrine, a physician is not liable if he or she provides care without parental consent when the care is within mainstream medical care, entails minimal risk, and is provided non-negligently, and the minor receiving care demonstrates maturity and decision-making capacity to consent to care and does consent voluntarily [5, 6]. Health professionals might rely on the mature minor doctrine, along with the constitutional right to privacy (discussed below), as justification for accepting the consent of mature minors seeking contraceptive services when state minor consent laws do not contain explicit authorization for a minor to consent.

Providers should review the laws in their own state to develop a clear understanding of when minors may consent to contraceptive services; providers may also wish to consult health care lawyers or professional medical organizations to clarify the law, especially since court decisions can sometimes affect the interpretation of statutes.

Federal Laws

Along with state laws, federal law supports a minor's ability to consent to contraceptive services. The United States Supreme Court has ruled that the constitutional right to privacy encompasses minors' reproductive decisions, including a minor's access to contraceptive services [5, 7]. Courts have rejected laws which attempted to explicitly require parental consent or notification for contraceptives [1, 5]. Given these legal findings, adolescent health law expert Abigail English suggests that "even in the absence of a statute that authorizes minors to consent for family planning services or contraceptive care, if there is no valid statute or case prohibiting them from doing so, it would be reasonable to conclude that minors may give their own consent for these services," further noting that this conclusion would be consistent with the mature minor doctrine [5].

Federal programs, such as Medicaid and the Title X Family Planning Program, also contain provisions that allow minors to access contraceptive services. Title X is a federal grant program designed to provide access to contraceptive services, supplies, and information to all who want and need them, with a focus on serving low-income individuals. Title X guidelines specify that clinics receiving funding must provide family planning services without regard to age. The guidelines encourage family communication, but do not require it for a minor to receive services [8]. Thus, minors who visit sites that receive Title X funds are able to obtain family planning services and contraceptive care without parental consent or notification [1, 9]. Medicaid provides health insurance coverage for low-income women and adolescents, including coverage for "family planning services." Medicaid rules require confidential family planning services be made available to sexually active minors of child-bearing age who desire them and are eligible for the program [9–11]. Courts have invalidated mandates that would require parental consent or disclosure to parents when minors receive family planning services through Title X or Medicaid, since such requirements would conflict with the provisions requiring confidential care and access [12, 13]. A significant number of states have expanded Medicaid coverage by implementing family planning "waiver" programs that enable states to provide family planning services to women and adolescents who would otherwise not be eligible [14].

CONFIDENTIALITY AND CONTRACEPTIVE CARE FOR ADOLESCENTS

The laws which authorize minors to consent to contraceptive care on their own do not always settle questions of confidentiality regarding that treatment. Rules governing the provision of confidential care for a minor stem from federal and state laws, regulations, and professional practice.

Studies have shown that adolescents' concerns about confidential care regarding reproductive health and contraceptive services can play an important role in their willingness to seek care [15]; in particular, concerns can lead them to delay or forgo care [2, 3, 16–18], affect their choice of provider [19], and impact their willingness to candidly disclose sensitive information [20]. Studies have also shown that delays and foregone care associated with the loss of confidentiality may result in higher rates of teen pregnancy and STIs, along with associated economic costs [17, 18, 21, 22].

Given the importance of confidential care for minors seeking reproductive health services, numerous leading professional medical organizations, including the Society for Adolescent Medicine, the American Academy of Pediatrics, the American Congress of Obstetricians and Gynecologists, the American Academy of Family Physicians, and the American Public Health Association, support confidential care for adolescent patients while also encouraging family communication and compliance with the law [23]. This section will discuss some of the key laws and considerations regarding the provision of confidential contraceptive care for minors.

State Laws

In many states, laws which authorize minor consent also contain provisions that address confidentiality or disclosure of health information [1]. Separate state laws can also provide guidance on the circumstances when disclosure is required, permitted, or prohibited. These laws can come in the form of broader medical privacy laws which govern disclosure of health information or laws mandating reports of child abuse or neglect.

In some states, a general disclosure provision applies to all minor consent laws. For example, in a few states, the laws specify that, when a minor has consented to care on their own, information about that care cannot be shared without permission of the minor [1]. In other states, a disclosure provision may apply to one or more of the minor consent laws; for instance, state laws may authorize a minor to consent for a service such as testing for sexually transmitted infection and also contain language about whether disclosure is permitted regarding testing, diagnosis, and treatment. As a result, disclosure rules may vary from service to service even within a state. Most of the disclosure provisions address circumstances under which a health care provider may or may not disclose information to a parent or guardian when a minor has consented to care [1]. Providers working with minors should review their state laws for these rules on disclosure, which will also be relevant to understanding application of the Health Insurance Portability and Accountability Act (HIPAA) Privacy Rule.

Special Circumstances that May Require Breach of Confidentiality

Other laws shape confidential communications between providers and adolescent patients. Providers must follow state laws regarding public health reporting of communicable diseases, which include sexually-transmitted infections. State mandatory reporting laws require health care professionals to breach confidentiality in order to report suspicions of child abuse and neglect, including sexual abuse. Legal precedents also require disclosure in situations where a minor is presenting a serious risk of harm to self, including suicidal ideation or homicidal threats [24, 25]. Laws which specify when sexual activity with a minor or between minors is illegal can affect the practice of health professionals who provide contraceptive care to adolescents. These laws, often known as statutory rape laws, vary greatly from state to state, though every state criminalizes sex with a minor under a certain age. State laws often differ based on the age of the "victim" and the age difference between the victim and the "perpetrator" [25, 26]. The requirement to report statutory rape is determined by a state's definition of "child abuse"; guidelines on when a provider must report are often found in the section of the state's statutes that address child abuse [26].

In addressing the issue of mandatory reporting of sexual activity and abuse, a position paper from the American Academy of Family Physicians, the American Academy of Pediatrics, the American Congress of Obstetricians and Gynecologists, and the Society for Adolescent Health and Medicine recognizes that adolescent sexual activity is not necessarily synonymous with sexual abuse. The authors assert that sexually active adolescents should receive appropriate care and counseling, on a confidential basis if necessary. While affirming that providers must know their state laws and report cases of abuse, the authors observe that most reportable cases of sexual abuse and coercion can be identified through careful clinical assessment and they support laws which affirm the authority of health care professionals to exercise appropriate clinical judgment in reporting cases of sexual activity [25].

Federal Laws
HIPAA Privacy Rule
Pursuant to the Health Insurance Portability and Accountability Act of 1996 (HIPAA), the Department of Health and Human Services (HHS) issued regulations addressing access to and disclosure of confidential medical information. These regulations are embodied in what is known as the HIPAA Privacy Rule, which applies to entities such as health care providers and insurers, collectively referred to as "covered entities". Among other things, the HIPAA Privacy Rule establishes guidelines regarding disclosure of "protected health information" for any patient who is able to consent to his or her own care. Generally, the HIPAA Privacy Rule

prohibits a covered entity from disclosing an individual's protected health information without authorization from the individual, except for the purposes of treatment, payment, the entity's health care operations, or for specified public health purposes [12].

The HIPAA Privacy Rule contains particular provisions that apply to minors. For the purposes of HIPAA, parents or guardians are generally considered to be the "personal representatives" of unemancipated minors. As personal representatives, parents may exercise any rights under the Privacy Rule regarding the minor's protected health information, including accessing that information [12]. However, if a minor is considered an "individual" under the Privacy Rule, then parents are not automatically treated as personal representatives. There are three situations when a minor may be considered an "individual": (1) when the minor has the legal right to consent to care and has consented; (2) when the minor may legally receive care without the consent of a parent, and the minor (or a third party such as a court) has consented; or (3) when a parent has assented to an agreement of confidentiality between the minor and the health care provider [12]. In each of these cases, the minor is treated as the "individual" who may exercise rights under the Privacy Rule and parents are not the personal representatives of the minor, unless the minor chooses to have them act in that capacity.

When a minor is the "individual" and a parent is not the personal representative, the minor may exercise most of the same rights as an adult under the HIPAA regulations. However, a parent who is not the personal representative of the minor may still have access to the minor's protected health information in some cases, as the HIPAA Privacy Rule defers to state or other applicable law on this question [12, 27, 28]. The relevant sources of state or other law include the following: state minor consent laws, state medical privacy laws, confidentiality rules for Medicaid and the Title X Family Planning Program; the federal confidentiality rules for drug or alcohol programs; and court cases interpreting these laws and the constitutional right of privacy [1]. As discussed above, state minor consent laws will often include some guidance on confidentiality or rules for disclosure. Some state medical records or medical privacy laws specifically provide confidentiality protection when minors are allowed to consent to their own care. Furthermore, professional licensing laws sometimes incorporate by reference the ethical codes of professional organizations, which can include confidentiality requirements [9].

If state or other laws explicitly require, permit, or prohibit disclosure of information to a parent, those laws are controlling, rather than the HIPAA Privacy Rule. For example, if a state or other law permits, but does not require, information to be disclosed to a parent, the regulations allow a health care provider to exercise discretion to disclose or not [12]. If a state law prohibits disclosure of information to a parent without the consent of a minor, the regulations do not allow a health care provider to disclose it without the minor's permission. When state laws do not provide any guidance on disclosure, under the HIPAA Privacy Rule, a licensed health care provider using professional judgment has discretion to determine whether to grant access for a parent, even in situations where the minor is able to consent to care on their own [12]. Providers working with adolescents seeking confidential care should be aware of this interplay between the HIPAA Privacy Rule and their own state laws.

Other Confidentiality Considerations
In addition to HIPAA, other federal rules have the potential to affect confidentiality. The Family Education Rights and Privacy Act (FERPA) allows parents to access a minor child's education records and the HIPAA Privacy Rule specifies that information covered by FERPA is not considered protected health information [12]. Issues regarding confidentiality protections may arise when adolescents receive care in a school-based health center (SBHC) or if health professionals employed by schools maintain student health records. However, it is usually the case that records in a SBHC would not be considered part of a student's educational record since they are often not administered by the school [12].

Certain requirements attached to federal programs, including Medicaid and Title X, contain specific confidentiality protections for minors receiving care through these programs. In particular, Title X guidelines require that providers encourage family participation, but Title X programs also must provide services without regard to age. Furthermore, all information about individuals receiving services "must be held confidential and must not be disclosed without the individual's documented consent" unless necessary to provide services or as required by law [8]. Legal requirements for disclosure include state laws requiring notification or reporting of child abuse, child molestation, sexual abuse, rape, or incest. Medicaid laws also require provision of confidential care for those who are eligible for the program, which includes coverage for family planning services [10, 11].

Adolescents with and without insurance coverage seek contraceptive care at Title X clinics, in part because of confidentiality protections. Even though many adolescents have insurance coverage, those seeking confidential care may not want to use their insurance to pay for services if documentation of the services (e.g., an explanation of benefits) will be sent to the policy holder, who is likely a parent or guardian. Under the HIPAA Privacy Rule, a minor using insurance acting as an "individual" may request that providers and health care plans communicate with him or her in a confidential manner (e.g., email or personal cell phone). He or she can also request that the information disclosed for treatment, payment, or other services be limited. However, there may be administrative hurdles to implementing such a plan unless there are effective protocols in place for both providers' offices and third-party payers [12]. Minors seeking assured confidentiality and affordability may turn to clinics funded by Title X, where patients are charged a sliding-scale fee based on the patient's—not the family's—income [8].

CONCLUSION

Given the complex framework of laws authorizing minor consent for contraceptive services and establishing confidentiality protections, health care providers serving adolescents should be knowledgeable about the laws and regulations governing their practice. Providers should develop standardized office policies and protocols for staff, patients, and parents regarding consent and confidentiality. Considering the important role that confidentiality plays for minors seeking health care, these policies and protocols should include information regarding the scope and limitations of confidentiality, guidelines for payment of services, medical chart access, appointment scheduling, and information disclosure [29].

REFERENCES

1. English A, Bass L, Dame Boyle A, Eshragh F. State minor consent laws: a summary. 3rd ed. Chapel Hill: Center for Adolescent Health & the Law; 2010.
2. Jones RK, Boonstra H. Confidential reproductive health services for minors: the potential impact of mandated parental involvement for contraception. Perspect Sex Reprod Health. 2004;36(5):182–91.
3. Jones RK, Purcell A, Singh S, Finer LB. Adolescents' reports of parental knowledge of adolescents' use of sexual health services and their reactions to mandated parental notification for prescription contraception. JAMA. 2005;293(3):340–8.
4. State policies in brief: minors' access to contraceptive services. New York: Guttmacher Institute. http://www.guttmacher.org/state-center/spibs/spib_MACS.pdf. Accessed 1 Feb 2013.
5. English A. Sexual and reproductive health care for adolescents: legal rights and policy challenges. Adolesc Med. 2007;18(3): 571–81.

6. Berlan E. Confidentiality, consent, and caring for the adolescent patient. Curr Opin Pediatr. 2009;21(4):450–6.
7. Carey v. Population Services International, 431 U.S. 678 (1977).
8. 42 U.S.C. § 300 et Seq. 42 CFR Part 59; Program guidelines for project grants for family planning services. Bethesda: United States Department of Health and Human Services, Office of Public Health and Science, Office of Population Affairs, Office of Family Planning. 2001. http://www.hhs.gov/opa/pdfs/2001-ofp-guidelines.pdf
9. Center for Adolescent Health & the Law; Healthy Teen Network. Confidential contraceptive services for adolescents: what health care providers need to know about the law. 2006. http://www.cahl.org/PDFs/HelpingTeensStayHealthy&Save_Full%20Report.pdf. Accessed 20 Mar 2012.
10. 42 U.S.C. § 1396d(a)(4)(C).
11. 42 U.S.C. § 1396a(a)(7).
12. English A, Ford CA. The HIPAA privacy rule and adolescents: legal questions and clinical challenges. Perspect Sex Reprod Health. 2004;36(2):80–6.
13. E.g., T.H. v. Jones, 425 F. Supp. 873 (D. Utah 1975), aff'd, 425 U.S. 986 (1976) (finding violation of Supremacy Clause and Fourteenth Amendment); County of St. Charles, Missouri v. Missouri Family Health Council, 107 F. 3d 682, 684–85 (8th Cir. 1997); Planned Parenthood Ass'n v. Dandoy, 810 F.2d 984, 986–88 (10th Cir. 1987); Jane Does 1 through 4 v. Utah Dep't of Health, 776 F.2d 253, 255 (10th Cir. 1985); New York v. Heckler, 719 F.2d 1191, 1196 (2d Cir. 1983); Planned Parenthood Fed'n v. Heckler, 712 F.2d 650, 656–63 (D.C. Cir. 1983).
14. Guttmacher Institute. State policies in brief: Medicaid family planning eligibility expansions. New York: Guttmacher Institute; 2012.
15. English A, Ford CA. More evidence supports the need to protect confidentiality in adolescent health care. J Adolesc Health. 2007;40(3):199–200.
16. Zabin LS, Stark HA, Emerson MR. Reasons for delay in contraceptive clinic utilization: adolescent clinic and nonclinic populations compared. J Adolesc Health. 1991;12(3):225–32.
17. Reddy DM, Fleming R, Swain C. Effect of mandatory parental notification on adolescent girls' use of sexual health care services. JAMA. 2002;288(6):710–4.
18. Lehrer JA, Pantell R, Tebb K, Shafer M-A. Forgone health care among U.S. adolescents: associations between risk characteristics and confidentiality concern. J Adolesc Health. 2007;40(3):218–26.
19. Sugerman S, Halfon N, Fink A, Anderson M, Valle L, Brook RH. Family planning clinic patients: their usual health care providers, insurance status, and implications for managed care. J Adolesc Health. 2000;27(1):25–33.

20. Ford CA, Millstein SG, Halpern-Felsher BL, Irwin CE. Influence of physician confidentiality assurances on adolescents' willingness to disclose information and seek future health care. JAMA. 1997; 278(12):1029–34.
21. Zavodny M. Fertility and parental consent for minors to receive contraceptives. Am J Public Health. 2004;94(8):1347–51.
22. Franzini L, Marks E, Cromwell PF, Risser J, McGill L, Markham C, et al. Projected economic costs due to health consequences of teenagers' loss of confidentiality in obtaining reproductive health care services in Texas. Arch Pediatr Adolesc Med. 2004;158(12): 1140–6.
23. Morreale M, Stinnett A, Dowling E. Policy compendium on confidential health services for adolescents. Chapel Hill, NC: Center for Adolescent Health & the Law; 2005.
24. Ford C, English A, Sigman G. Confidential health care for adolescents: position paper of the society for adolescent medicine. J Adolesc Health. 2004;35(2):160–7.
25. Position paper of the American Academy of Family Physicians, The American Academy of Pediatrics, The American College of Obstetricians and Gynecologists, and The Society for Adolescent Medicine. Protecting adolescents: ensuring access to care and reporting sexual activity and abuse. J Adolesc Health: official publication of the Society for Adolescent Medicine. 2004;35(5):420–3.
26. Dailard C. Statutory rape reporting and family planning programs: moving beyond conflict. The Guttmacher Report on Public Policy. 2004;7(2):10–2.
27. Rosenbaum S, Abramson S, MacTaggart P. Health information law in the context of minors. Pediatrics. 2009;123 Suppl 2:S116–21.
28. 45 CFR 160 and 164.
29. Access to health care for adolescents and young adults: Position paper of the Society for Adolescent Medicine. J Adolesc Health 2004;35(4):342–4.

Chapter 14
Pregnancy Options Counseling

Stephanie Sober and Courtney A. Schreiber

DEMOGRAPHICS/SCOPE
Unintended Pregnancy

Half of all US pregnancies are unintended [1]. In the United States, unintended pregnancy rates are higher among women aged 18–24 [1]. The proportion of pregnancies that are unintended generally decreases as age increases. The highest unintended pregnancy rate in 2006 was among women aged 20–24 (107 per 1,000 women) [1]. Of the approximately 750,000 pregnancies that occur among teens every year, more than 80 % are unintended [2]. Thus, teens account for almost one-fifth of all unintended pregnancies [1]. Calculations of the unintended pregnancy rate typically include all women, whether or not they are sexually active. Since many teens are not sexually active, the rate among teens is actually understated [3]. The unintended pregnancy rate among only sexually active teens is more than twice the rate among all women.

Pregnancy Resolution

Barring any major changes in the US abortion rate, 30 % of women will have an abortion by age 45, 25 % of women will have an abortion by age 30, and 8 % by age 20 [4]. More than half of American women obtaining abortions are in their 20s, and women aged 20–24 have the highest abortion rate of any age group (40 abortions

S. Sober, M.D. • C.A. Schreiber, M.D., M.P.H. (✉)
Department of Obstetrics and Gynecology, Hospital of the University
of Pennsylvania, 3400 Spruce Street, 1000 Courtyard, Philadelphia,
PA 19104, USA
e-mail: stephanie.sober1@uphs.upenn.edu; cschreiber@obgyn.upenn.edu

A. Whitaker and M. Gilliam (eds.), *Contraception for Adolescent*
and Young Adult Women, DOI 10.1007/978-1-4614-6579-9_14,
© Springer Science+Business Media New York 2014

per 1,000 women per year) [4]. Teenagers account for just 17 % of all US abortions [5]. Teens aged 18–19 account for 11 % of all abortions, and 15–17-year-olds account for 6 %; teens younger than age 15 account for only 0.4 %. Thus, teens aged 18–19 obtain two out of three teen abortions. There are 19 abortions for every 1,000 women aged 15–19 in the United States per year [2]. The abortion rate is higher than average for black and Hispanic teens (44 and 24 per 1,000 women aged 15–19, respectively) and lower than average for non-Hispanic white teens (11 per 1,000). However, the majority (nearly 60 %) of US teen pregnancies end in birth, while 27 % end in abortion, and the remainder end in miscarriage [2]. Only 2 % of unmarried pregnant women at any age place their child for adoption [6]. The proportion of teens placing their children for adoption has declined over recent decades with less than 1 % choosing this option [6].

PREGNANCY OPTIONS COUNSELING
Pregnancy options counseling should be unbiased, nonjudgmental, and nondirective [7, 8]. The counselor should provide medically accurate and factual information about all options available including pregnancy continuation, prenatal care and delivery, adoption, and abortion in order to help the woman come to the decision that is best for her. The counseling session should be conducted in a supportive manner in a safe, confidential setting. An effective counselor will help a woman explore her feelings about pregnancy, her values, resources, and plans for the future (see sample questions from Pregnancy Options Workbook) (Table 14.1). The counselor helps a woman prepare for how her choice may affect her relationships, goals, and sense of well-being. According to the Title X guidelines, nondirective counseling should "help clients resolve uncertainty, ambivalence, and anxiety in relation to reproductive health and to enhance their capacity to arrive at a decision that reflects their considered self-interest" [9].

Abortion
The discussion should include a factual description of the various abortion methods available including medication abortion (if appropriate) as well as surgical or vacuum aspiration. The counselor should discuss what to expect in general—prior to, during, and after the procedure—and address any specific questions or concerns of the patient. The counselor should encourage the patient to discuss her feelings about abortion and to seek support resources if necessary.

TABLE 14.1 Examples of questions for patients to think about [23].

- Do I want to have a baby?

- Will the child have a father who is "there"?

- Can I afford to have a child?

- What will happen to my goals, my hopes, my life?

- What will happen to my partner's life?

- Who can help me raise a child?

- Can I raise a child by myself?

- How will my family react? My friends?

- How will this affect my other children?

- Is my body healthy enough?

- In other words: IS THIS THE RIGHT TIME FOR ME TO BE RESPONSIBLE FOR A CHILD?

From: Pregnancy Options Workbook, www.pregnancyoptions.info; with permission

Prenatal Care and Parenting

The discussion should include information on prenatal care, labor and delivery, as well as infant care. The counselor should discuss what to expect in general and address any specific questions or concerns of the patient. The counselor should also encourage a realistic discussion of whether a child would fit into the patient's life, whether the patient is financially ready to have a child, and whether she has enough support from family members or others for all that is involved in raising a child.

Prenatal Care and Adoption

The discussion should include a reminder that all of the information regarding prenatal care, labor, and delivery reviewed during the parenting discussion would also apply in this scenario. The patient should understand the definition of adoption, which legally means surrendering her right to parent her child and giving someone else the permission to take on the legal right and responsibility of parenting her child. She should be advised about the distinction between "agency" adoption and "private" adoption through an adoption lawyer as well as the various types of adoption, including open (able to have contact with adoptive parents and the child), semi-open (contact through adoption agency or lawyer), and closed (no contact) adoptions. She should understand that she will be able to choose which option she prefers.

Box 14.1   The Pregnancy Options Workbook letter to reader

Dear Reader,

If this workbook is in your hands, you are probably pregnant and not sure what to do. You're in the right place. Read on. The people who put together this book support you no matter what you choose. We have tried to give you a realistic picture of all the choices you can make—abortion, adoption, and being a parent. You will find exercises to help you make the best decision for you. We have also included information and thoughts on Religion and Spirituality, Fetal Development, and What Can Harm A Pregnancy. There is a special section called Taking Care of Yourself which includes information on morning sickness, birth control, protecting your fertility, and healthy sexuality.

If you are having a hard time with your decision, you may think you can never feel good about your choice. We have found that women who are willing to explore what they think and how they feel can come to a peaceful resolution. To get there, you must be willing to work at it. So, get out your crayons, sharpen your pencils, and do some "homework." It may be the most important homework you ever do. Remember to listen to your heart and your own voice to find the right answer for you. Get some help if you need it.

Thank you and Good Luck!

From: Pregnancy Options Workbook, www.pregnancyoptions. info; with permission

An exceptional resource for patients of all ages, but particularly useful for adolescents and young adults, is the Pregnancy Options Workbook (can be found online at www.pregnancyoptions.info). This workbook guides the woman through exercises designed to help her explore her feelings about the pregnancy in order to help her make the right decision for her (see letter to readers from Pregnancy Options Workbook) (Box 14.1). The workbook encourages women to find sources of support and also provides resources for how to discuss the situation with partners and family members (including specific cutout pages for male partners and parents). The workbook includes sections with comprehensive information on each of the three options as well as resources and referrals for patients choosing each option.

Pregnancy options counseling does not—and should not—involve advocacy of any one option. It is especially important for the counselor to identify and understand her own values and beliefs when conducting pregnancy options counseling (particularly with adolescents). The patient must be able to make decisions that will make sense for her life, based on her own beliefs. Access to full information and freedom from coercion is crucial. To that end, each woman should initially be interviewed alone for at least a portion of the counseling session in order to afford her the opportunity to disclose coercion by her family members or partner. Key steps in pregnancy options counseling include:

- Ask the patient how she feels.
- Allow the patient time to process and speak about her feelings. In pregnancy options counseling, how a patient feels will drive her decision. During the counseling session, use of a needs assessment form can sometimes assist in determining the patient's emotional status (Chap. 14 Appendix).
- Present all options without neglecting or overly emphasizing any single option.
- Make sure the patient knows what her options are and that any misconceptions about her options are addressed.

The counseling session helps the patient get a clear picture of how she feels about being pregnant so that she can make the right decision for her given her life circumstances, values, and desires. The decision absolutely has to be that of the pregnant woman, made freely, without coercion from others. Once she decides how to proceed, the counselor can refer her for the services requested, which may include additional counseling if so desired. Perhaps best stated by some of the experts in the field, "Appropriate, sensitive communication that focuses on the needs of each patient is fundamental to quality care... The key to achieving effective clinician-patient communication is empathy—the ability to give the clear, comforting message that one is not superior to the patient but shares with her a common bond of humanity" [8].

Special Concerns for Adolescents
For some women, pregnancy options counseling may be an intensely emotional experience because of personal circumstances, ambivalence, or intense and perhaps conflicting feelings the decision evokes [7]. The adolescent, in particular, is facing many pressures already, and the counseling session must offer her a safe place in which to explore her feelings freely. The decision is difficult for the adolescent who has not yet completed her individuation and thus is not accustomed to making autonomous

choices [10]. If the adolescent is still living at home, she may be controlled by her parents' decisions, either to please them or because she requires their ongoing financial or emotional support. When possible, parental support should be sought and the family helped to deal with the event together. She may want to talk about whether to inform the father of her pregnancy or to involve him in her decision making.

It is particularly important to be direct and concrete with adolescents as their ability to understand the concept of consequence is still in development [10]. The adolescent should be encouraged to talk about her knowledge of pregnancy and her ideas about the course of pregnancy and how she imagines she will feel. Discussions about the delivery and care of the newborn are important as well as the constraints on her time and actions because of child care. Financial needs and the expenses involved in parenting must also be addressed in a direct, concrete manner. Practical issues such as where she can live during and after the pregnancy, whether she will remain in school or at a job, and how her friends and family will react should be discussed. The adolescent's feelings about adoption and abortion as options must also be explored. If she is considering abortion, the possible procedures should be fully explained in a matter-of-fact manner. Any legal issues applicable in her home state must be outlined, as well as any need for parental consent or notification [11].

The counselor's role is to enable the adolescent to explore and resolve any ambivalence she may have about the course and outcome of the pregnancy and to reach a decision with which she is comfortable. The counselor should assist the patient in evaluating the importance she places on school, employment, socialization, and family relationships and how she believes a pregnancy would affect all of this—as well as how it would affect the rest of her life. In addition, the adolescent should be encouraged to talk about her sexuality, becoming pregnant, and future sexual behavior. Contraceptive advice and information should be given to her at this time if appropriate. Finally, she should be told about support resources should she need them during the pregnancy and postpartum or after an abortion. According to Gold [10], "we must offer teenagers the benefit of our knowledge, reasoned unbiased counsel, and, when necessary, therapy suitable to their developmental status."

Parental Involvement and the Law

The majority of states have laws that require parents to consent to or be notified of a minor's decision to have an abortion. Specifically, 37 states require some type of parental involvement in a minor's decision to have an abortion: 21 states require one or both parents to consent to the procedure, 11 require that one or both parents be notified, and 5 states require both parental consent and notification [12]. However, due to the Supreme Court ruling that states may not give parents absolute veto power over their daughter's decision, most state parental involvement requirements include a judicial bypass procedure that allows the minor to receive court approval for an abortion without her parents' knowledge or consent. Many parental involvement requirements are waived in cases of medical emergency or if the minor is the victim of abuse or neglect [13]. The Guttmacher Institute website lists each specific state's parental notification requirements. Laws requiring parental involvement in minors' abortion decisions appear to do little to reduce teen abortion or pregnancy rates [14]. These laws do, however, serve as barriers, delaying access to the procedure, thereby reducing safety and resulting in later abortions.

Family Involvement
The adolescent should be encouraged to include parents and the partner in these counseling sessions [15]. The provider can often help the adolescent patient plan an optimum way of telling her parent(s) that may include the mediating presence of another family member. The website www.MomDadIMpregnant.com [16] is an extremely helpful resource for both adolescents and parents. However, if the patient is a minor, the provider must seek assurance that she is not being coerced by her parent(s). Only when it is clear that parental coercion is not a factor should the provider obtain any government-mandated parental consent or notification or the consent of a court and secure the appropriate forms for the medical record [7]. When an adolescent predicts severe repercussions or is otherwise unable or unwilling to involve a parent, the provider can help the patient navigate the judicial bypass process. Providers in the United States, as well as local attorneys, can contact the American Civil Liberties Union Reproductive Freedom Project for guidance on the judicial bypass process. If parental support is not possible, minors should be advised to seek the advice and counsel of adults they trust, including other relatives, counselors, teachers, or clergy. This is especially true for younger adolescents, age 12–15 years [15]. It is important to identify the patient's support system as it is crucial that adolescents have support while making their decision.

Sexual Abuse/Incest
If the adolescent is reluctant to reveal the identity of the man with whom she became pregnant, the counselor should consider the possibility of sexual abuse, sexual assault, or incest. Counselors should be aware of state laws about reporting suspected abuse or statutory rape and take appropriate action [15]. As stated above, it

is imperative to talk with the adolescent alone at some point in the counseling process to allow an opportunity for disclosure of any confidential information that she may not be free to discuss in the presence of other people.

Adolescents' Coping/Mental Health

Although some studies suggest that adolescence is a potential risk factor for negative emotional sequelae after abortion, longitudinal research shows that adolescents do not have a higher incidence of negative reactions, such as long-term regret or depression [17]. In the short-term, teens may be more likely to engage in avoidant coping methods such as denial and mental disengagement and have less confidence in their ability to cope successfully with the abortion than adults. However, by 2 years postabortion, these age-group differences in adjustment disappear [17]. Another study of US teens who have had an abortion shows that this group is not at higher risk for depression or low self-esteem than teens who carry their pregnancy to term [18]. Similarly, studies indicate a lack of negative mental health effects of abortion among adult women.

For adolescents, the reactions of parents can significantly increase or reduce emotional distress. Research has found that negative, antagonistic, or conditional support from parents is more detrimental to a young woman's postabortion psychological adjustment than the absence of disclosure [19]. When someone other than the adolescent herself discloses the pregnancy to her parents, the likelihood of a negative outcome increases [20]. Furthermore, the adolescent who chooses not to tell her parents, but believes they would be supportive of her decision, copes better after abortion than the adolescent who tells her parents but receives less than full support [20–22]. Thus, the prospect of parental involvement should be discussed thoroughly with each patient in an attempt to determine whether it will be beneficial to the patient on an individual basis. Unfortunately, there is no appreciable literature regarding the mental health of adolescents who choose either parenting or adoption.

In summary, the young woman has the responsibility to weigh the risks and benefits of abortion versus parenting versus adoption and choose the option that is most appropriate in light of her personal values, relationships, and goals. All pregnancy-related outcomes are benefited by early diagnosis and management. She should be counseled to consider all options, encouraged to return for as many visits as needed, and helped to understand the need to make a timely decision. She should also be reminded that this decision is never easy, and that, in the words of the Pregnancy Options Workbook, "all decisions about pregnancy require some sacrifice."

RESOURCES

Effective resources for patients who need spiritual support can be found at www.faithaloud.org, http://cath4choice.org, www.hope-clinic.org, and www.pregnancyoptions.info

If the patient can identify no one she can trust, then offering her a referral for postabortion phone counseling can supply accessible, confidential, and nonjudgmental support—www.4exhale.org or www.yourbackline.org

The Pregnancy Options Workbook: www.pregnancyoptions.info
Abortion Care Network: www.MomDadIMpregnant.com

APPENDIX: Sample needs assessment form[a]. [a]Courtesy of Penn Family Planning and Pregnancy Loss Center.

PFPPLC Needs Assessment   Affix Label Here

To participate with you in your care and give you proper support, we need to know if you agree or disagree with the following statements at this time. Please answer these questions honestly so that we can work together to maximize your emotional and physical care.

I am sure about my decision to terminate this pregnancy.
Strongly agree ☐   Agree ☐   Neither agree nor disagree ☐   Disagree ☐   Strongly disagree ☐

Someone else is pushing me to terminate this pregnancy.
Strongly agree ☐   Agree ☐   Neither agree nor disagree ☐   Disagree ☐   Strongly disagree ☐

Who is pushing you to terminate? (Circle all that are true)
My Mom	Boyfriend	Husband	The man that got me pregnant
Aunt	My Father	Everybody	Grandmother
Friend	My Doctor	Other_____	

I wish I could carry this pregnancy to term.
Strongly agree ☐   Agree ☐   Neither agree nor disagree ☐   Disagree ☐   Strongly disagree ☐

Generally after making a decision, I doubt myself.
Strongly agree ☐   Agree ☐   Neither agree nor disagree ☐   Disagree ☐   Strongly disagree ☐

At this time, terminating the pregnancy is the best choice for me:
Strongly agree ☐   Agree ☐   Neither agree nor disagree ☐   Disagree ☐   Strongly disagree ☐

Today I am feeling:

	Not at all	A little bit	Moderate	Quite a bit	Extremely
Calm					
Confident					
Relieved					
Sick					
Nervous					
Scared					
Angry					
Ashamed					
Sad					
Guilty					

Other_____

I have or have had: (Circle all that are true)
Depression	Anxiety	Panic Attacks	Bipolar Disorder
ADD	Schizophrenia	Eating disorder	
Borderline Personality Disorder			

Who knows about this pregnancy termination? (Please circle any that are true for you)
My Mom	Boyfriend	Husband	The man that got me pregnant
Aunt	My Father	Everybody	Grandmother
Friend(s)	Neighbor(s)	Workplace	
Other_____			

DOUBLE SIDED, please turn OVER—→   06/2010

APPENDIX: (continued)

PFPPLC Needs Assessment   Affix Label Here

The people I have told about this decision are supportive of me.
Strongly agree ☐   Agree ☐   Neither agree nor disagree ☐   Disagree ☐   Strongly disagree ☐

(If you have had a termination in the past): I did emotionally well after the termination.
Strongly agree ☐   Agree ☐   Neither agree nor disagree ☐   Disagree ☐   Strongly disagree ☐
Never had termination in the past ☐

I have some spiritual concerns about this termination.
Strongly agree ☐   Agree ☐   Neither agree nor disagree ☐   Disagree ☐   Strongly disagree ☐

After the procedure, I think I will feel:

	Not at all	A little bit	Moderate	Quite a bit	Extremely
Calm					
Confident					
Relieved					
Pain					
Nervous					
Scared					
Angry					
Ashamed					
Sad					
Guilty					
Other					

How do you think you'll deal with your feelings after the procedure? (Circle any that are true for you)
   I'll be fine afterwards
   It'll be a little hard, but I'll be fine afterwards
   It will be VERY hard for me to deal with this
   I'll wish I'd never done this
   I will cope with this decision better than if I had carried the pregnancy to term

Patient Signature:_____   Date:_____   Time:_____

Physician Signature:_____   Date:_____   Time:_____

06/2010

REFERENCES

1. Finer LB, Zolna MR. Unintended pregnancy in the United States: incidence and disparities. Contraception. 2011;84(5):478–85.
2. Kost K, Henshaw S, Carlin L. U.S. teenage pregnancies, births and abortions: national and state trends and trends by race and ethnicity. New York: Guttmacher Institute; 2010.
3. Finer LB. Unintended pregnancy among U.S. adolescents: accounting for sexual activity. J Adolesc Health. 2010;47(3):312–4.
4. Jones RK, Kavanaugh ML. Changes in abortion rates between 2000 and 2008 and lifetime incidence of abortion. Obstet Gynecol. 2011;117(6):1358–66.

5. Jones RK, Finer LB, Singh S. Characteristics of U.S. abortion patients, 2008. New York: Guttmacher Institute; 2010.
6. Moore KA, Miller BC, Sugland BW, Morrison DR, Glei DA, Blumenthal C. Beginning too soon: adolescent sexual behavior, pregnancy, and parenthood. Washington, DC: Child Trends, Inc.; 1995.
7. Baker A, Beresford T. Informed consent, patient education, and counseling. In: Paul M, Lichtenberg ES, Borgatta L, Grimes DA, Stubblefield PG, Creinin MD, editors. Management of unintended and abnormal pregnancy. 1st ed. Chichester, West Sussex: Wiley-Blackwell Publishing; 2009. p. 48–62.
8. Baker A, Beresford T, Halvorson-Boyd G, Garrity JM. Informed consent, counseling, and patient preparation. In: Paul M, Lichtenberg ES, Borgatta L, Grimes DA, Stubblefield PG, editors. A Clinician's guide to medical and surgical abortion. Philadelphia: Churchill Livingstone; 1999. p. 25–37.
9. Dailard C. Family planning and adoption promotion: new proposals, long-standing issues. Guttmacher Rep Public Policy. 1999; 2(5):1–13.
10. Gold JH. Adolescents and abortion. In: Stotland NL, editor. Psychiatric aspects of abortion. Washington, DC: American Psychiatric Press, Inc.; 1991. p. 187–95.
11. Gold RB, Nash E. State abortion counseling policies and the fundamental principles of informed consent. Guttmacher Policy Review. 2007;10(4):6–13.
12. Guttmacher Institute. An overview of abortion laws. State Policies in Brief (as of October 1, 2011). Cited 2012 March. http://www.guttmacher.org/statecenter/spibs/spib_OAL.pdf
13. Guttmacher Institute. Parental involvement in minors' abortions. State Policies in Brief (as of March 1, 2012). Cited 2012 March. http://www.guttmacher.org/statecenter/spibs/spib_PIMA.pdf
14. Dennis A, Henshaw SK, Joyce TJ, Finer LB, Blanchard K. The impact of laws requiring parental involvement for abortion: a literature review. New York: Guttmacher Institute; 2009.
15. American Academy of Pediatrics (AAP) Committee on Adolescence. Counseling the adolescent about pregnancy options. Pediatrics. 1998;101(5):938–40.
16. Abortion Care Network, www.MomDadIMpregnant.com
17. Quinton WJ, Major B, Richards C. Adolescents and adjustment to abortion: are minors at greater risk? Psychol Public Policy Law. 2001;7(3):491–514.
18. Warren JT, Harvey SM, Henderson JT. Do depression and low self-esteem follow abortion among adolescents? Evidence from a national study. Perspect Sex Reprod Health. 2010;42(4):230–5.
19. Griffen-Carlson MS, Schwanenflugel PJ. Adolescent abortion and parental notification: evidence for the importance of family functioning on the perceived quality of parental involvement in US families. J Child Psychol Psychiatry. 1998;39(4):543–53.

20. Major B, Cozzarelli C, Sciacchitano AM, Cooper ML, Testa M, Mueller PM. Perceived social support, self-efficacy, and adjustment to abortion. J Pers Soc Psychol. 1990;59(3):452–63.
21. Cozzarelli C. Personality and self-efficacy as predictors of coping with abortion. J Pers Soc Psychol. 1993;65(6):1224–36.
22. Major B, Richards C, Cooper ML, Cozzarelli C, Zubeck J. Personal resilience, cognitive appraisals, and coping: an integrative model of adjustment to abortion. J Pers Soc Psychol. 1998;74(3):735–52.
23. Pregnancy Options Workbook, www.pregnancyoptions.info

Appendix A
Categories of Medical Eligibility Criteria for Contraceptive Use

1	A condition for which there is no restriction for the use of the contraceptive method
2	A condition for which the advantages of using the method generally outweigh the theoretical or proven risks
3	A condition for which the theoretical or proven risks usually outweigh the advantages of using the method
4	A condition that represents an unacceptable health risk if the contraceptive method is used

Source: Centers for Disease Control and Prevention. U.S. medical eligibility criteria for contraceptive use, 2010. MMWR. 2010;59(RR-4):1–86.

A. Whitaker and M. Gilliam (eds.), *Contraception for Adolescent and Young Adult Women*, DOI 10.1007/978-1-4614-6579-9,
© Springer Science + Business Media New York 2014

Appendix B

Summary Chart of *US Medical Eligibility Criteria for Contraceptive Use, 2010*

 Updated June 2012. This summary sheet only contains a subset of the recommendations from the US MEC.

For complete guidance, see:
http://www.cdc.gov/reproductivehealth/
unintendedpregnancy/
USMEC.htm.

Most contraceptive methods do not protect against sexually transmitted infections (STIs). Consistent and correct use of the male latex condom reduces the risk of STIs and HIV.

Source: Centers for Disease Control and Prevention. U.S. medical eligibility criteria for contraceptive use, 2010. MMWR. 2010;59(RR-4):1–86.

A. Whitaker and M. Gilliam (eds.), *Contraception for Adolescent and Young Adult Women*, DOI 10.1007/978-1-4614-6579-9,
© Springer Science + Business Media New York 2014

Condition	Sub-condition	Combined pill, patch, ring		Progestin-only pill		Injection		Implant		LNG-IUD		Copper-IUD	
		I	C	I	C	I	C	I	C	I	C	I	C
Age		Menarche to <40 = 1 ≥40 = 2		Menarche to <18 = 1 18–45 = 1 >45 = 1		Menarche to <18 = 2 18–45 = 1 >45 = 2		Menarche to <18 = 1 18–45 = 1 >45 = 1		Menarche to <20 = 2 ≥20 = 1		Menarche to <20 = 2 ≥20 = 1	
Anatomic abnormalities	(a) Distorted uterine cavity									4		4	
	(b) Other abnormalities									2		2	
Anemias	(a) Thalassemia	1		1		1		1		1		2	
	(b) Sickle cell disease[a]	2		1		1		1		1		2	
	(c) Iron-deficiency anemia	1		1		1		1		1		2	
Benign ovarian tumors	(Including cysts)	1		1		1		1		1		1	
Breast disease	(a) Undiagnosed mass	2[b]		2[b]		2[b]		2[b]		2		1	
	(b) Benign breast disease	1		1		1		1		1		1	
	(c) Family history of cancer	1		1		1		1		1		1	
	(d) Breast cancer[a]												
	(i) Current	4		4		4		4		4		1	
	(ii) Past and no evidence of current disease for 5 years	3		3		3		3		3		1	

Breastfeeding (see also postpartum)	(a) <1 month postpartum	3[b]	2[b]	2[b]	2[b]			2
	(b) 1 month or more postpartum	2[b]	1[b]	1[b]	1[b]	1		
Cervical cancer	Awaiting treatment	2	1	2	2	4	2	2
Cervical ectropion		1	1	1	1	1		1
Cervical intraepithelial neoplasia		2	1	2	2	2		1
Cirrhosis	(a) Mild (compensated)	1	1	1	1	1		1
	(b) Severe[a] (decompensated)	4	3	3	3	3		1
DVT/PE	(a) History of DVT/PE, not on anticoagulant therapy							
	(i) Higher risk for recurrent DVT/PE	4	2	2	2	2		1
	(ii) Lower risk for recurrent DVT/PE	3	2	2	2	2		1
	(b) Acute DVT/PE	4	2	2	2	2		2
	(c) DVT/PE established on anticoagulant therapy for at least 3 months	2	2	2	2	2		

(continued)

(continued)

Condition	Sub-condition	Combined pill, patch, ring		Progestin-only pill		Injection		Implant		LNG-IUD		Copper-IUD	
		I	C	I	C	I	C	I	C	I	C	I	C
	(i) Higher risk for recurrent DVT/PE	4[b]		2		2		2		2		2	
	(ii) Lower risk for recurrent DVT/PE	3[b]		2		2		2		2		2	
	(d) Family history (first-degree relatives)	2		1		1		1		1		1	
	(e) Major surgery												
	(i) With prolonged immobilization	4		2		2		2		2		1	
	(ii) Without prolonged immobilization	2		1		1		1		1		1	
	(f) MINOR surgery without immobilization	1		1		1		1		1		1	
Depressive disorders		1[b]		1[b]		1[b]		1[b]		1[b]		1[b]	

Diabetes mellitus	(a) History of gestational diabetes mellitus only	1	1	1	1	1	1
	(b) Non-vascular disease						
	(i) Non-insulin dependent	2	2	2	2	2	1
	(ii) Insulin dependent[a]	2	2	2	2	2	1
	(c) Nephropathy/retinopathy/neuropathy[a]	3/4[b]	3	2	2	2	1
	(d) Other vascular disease or diabetes of >20 years' duration[a]	3/4[b]	3	2	2	2	1
Endometrial cancer[a]		1	1	1	1	4	4	2
Endometrial hyperplasia		1	1	1	1	1	1
Endometriosis		1	1	1	1	2	1
Epilepsy[a]	(See also drug interactions)	1[b]	1[b]	1[b]	1[b]	1	1

(continued)

(continued)

Condition	Sub-condition	Combined pill, patch, ring		Progestin-only pill		Injection		Implant		LNG-IUD		Copper-IUD	
		I	C	I	C	I	C	I	C	I	C	I	C
Gallbladder disease	(a) Symptomatic												
	(i) Treated by cholecystectomy	2		2		2		2		2		1	
	(ii) Medically treated	3		2		2		2		2		1	
	(iii) Current	3		2		2		2		2		1	
	(b) Asymptomatic	2		2		2		2		2		1	
Gestational trophoblastic disease	(a) Decreasing or undetectable ß-hCG levels	1		1		1		1		3		3	
	(b) Persistently elevated fi-hCG levels or malignant disease[a]	1		1		1		1		4		4	
Headaches	(a) Non-migrainous	1[b]	2[b]	1[b]	1[b]	1[b]	1[b]	1[b]	1[b]	1[b]	1[b]	1[b]	
	(b) Migraine												
	(i) Without aura, age <35	2[b]	3[b]	1[b]	2[b]	2[b]	2[b]	2[b]	2[b]	2[b]	2[b]	1[b]	
	(ii) Without aura, age ≥35	3[b]	4[b]	1[b]	2[b]	2[b]	2[b]	2[b]	2[b]	2[b]	2[b]	1[b]	
	(iii) With aura, any age	4[b]	4[b]	2[b]	3[b]	2[b]	3[b]	2[b]	3[b]	2[b]	3[b]	1[b]	

History of bariatric surgery[a]	(a) Restrictive procedures	1	1	1	1	1	1
	(b) Malabsorptive procedures	COCs: 3 / P/R: 1	3	1	1	1	1
History of cholestasis	(a) Pregnancy-related	2	1	1	1	1	1
	(b) Past COC-related	3	2	2	2	2	1
History of high blood pressure during pregnancy		2	1	1	1	1	1
History of pelvic surgery		1	1	1	1	1	1
HIV	High risk	1	1	1	1	2	2
	HIV infected (see also drug interactions)[a]	1b	1b	1b	1b	2	2
	AIDS (see also drug interactions)[a]	1b	1b	1b	3	2b / 3	2b / 2
	Clinically well on therapy	If on treatment, see drug interactions		2	3	2	2	2

(continued)

(continued)

Condition	Sub-condition	Combined pill, patch, ring		Progestin-only pill		Injection		Implant		LNG-IUD		Copper-IUD	
		I	C	I	C	I	C	I	C	I	C	I	C
Hyperlipidemias		2/3[b]		2[b]		2[b]		2[b]		2[b]		1[b]	
Hypertension	(a) Adequately controlled hypertension	3[b]		1[b]		2[b]		1[b]		1		1	
	(b) Elevated blood pressure levels (properly taken measurements)												
	(i) Systolic 140–159 or diastolic 90–99	3		1		2		1		1		1	
	(ii) Systolic ≥160 or diastolic ≥100[b]	4		2		3		2		2		1	
	(c) Vascular disease	4		2		3		2		2		1	
Inflammatory bowel disease	(Ulcerative colitis, Crohn's disease)	2/3[b]		2		2		1		1		1	
Ischemic heart disease[a]	Current history	4		2	3	3		2	3	2	3	1	

Liver tumors	(a) Benign						
	(i) FOCAL nodular hyperplasia	2	2	2	2	2	1
	(ii) Hepatocellular adenoma[a]	4	3	3	3	3	1
	(b) Malignant[a]	4	3	3	3	3	1
Malaria		1	1	1	1	1	1
Multiple risk factors for arterial cardiovascular disease	(Such as older age, smoking, diabetes and, hypertension)	3/4[b]	2[b]	3[b]	2[b]	2[b]	1
Obesity	(a) ≥30 kg/m² BMI	2	1	1	1	1	1
	(b) Menarche to <18 years and ≥30 kg/m² BMI	2	1	2	1	1	1
Ovarian cancer[a]		1	1	1	1	1	1
Parity	(a) Nulliparous	1	1	1	1	2	2
	(b) Parous	1	1	1	1	1	1
Past ectopic pregnancy		1	2	1	1	1	1

(continued)

(continued)

Condition	Sub-condition	Combined pill, patch, ring		Progestin-only pill		Injection		Implant		LNG-IUD		Copper-IUD	
		I	C	I	C	I	C	I	C	I	C	I	C
Pelvic inflammatory disease	(a) Past (assuming no current risk factors of STIs)												
	(i) With subsequent pregnancy	1		1		1		1		1	1	1	1
	(ii) Without subsequent pregnancy	1		1		1		1		2	2	2	2
	(b) Current	1		1		1		1		4	2[b]	4	2[b]
Peripartum cardiomyopathy[a]	(a) Normal or mildly impaired cardiac function												
	(i) <6 months	4		1		1		1		2		2	
	(ii) ≥6 months	3		1		1		1		2		2	
	(b) Moderately or severely impaired cardiac function	4		2		2		2		2		2	
Postabortion	(a) First trimester	1[b]		1[b]		1[b]		1[b]		1[b]		1[b]	
	(b) Second trimester	1[b]		1[b]		1[b]		1[b]		2		2	
	(c) Immediately post-septic abortion	1[b]		1[b]		1[b]		1[b]		4		4	

Postpartum (see also breastfeeding)						
(a) <21 days	4	1	1	1		
(b) 21–42 days						
(i) With other risk factors for VTE	3[b]	1	1	1		
(ii) Without other risk factors for VTE	2	1	1	1		
(c) >42 days	1	1	1	1		
Postpartum (in breastfeeding or non-breastfeeding women, including post-cesarean section)						
(a) <10 min after delivery of the placenta					2	1
(b) 10 min after delivery of the placenta to <4 weeks					2	2
(c) ≥4 weeks					1	1
(d) Puerperal sepsis					4	4
Pregnancy	NA[b]	NA[b]	NA[b]	NA[b]	4[b]	4[b]
Rheumatoid arthritis						
(a) On immunosuppressive therapy	2	2/3[b]	1	2	2	1
(b) Not on immunosuppressive therapy	2	2	1	1	1	1

(continued)

(continued)

Condition	Sub-condition	Combined pill, patch, ring		Progestin-only pill		Injection		Implant		LNG-IUD		Copper-IUD	
		I	C	I	C	I	C	I	C	I	C	I	C
Schistosomiasis	(a) Uncomplicated	1		1		1		1		1		1	
	(b) Fibrosis of the liver[a]	1		1		1		1		1		1	
Severe dysmenorrhea		1		1		1		1		1		2	
STIs	(a) Current purulent cervicitis or chlamydial infection or gonorrhea	1		1		1		1		4	2[b]	4	2[b]
	(b) Other STIs (excluding HIV and hepatitis)	1		1		1		1		2	2	2	2
	(c) Vaginitis (including trichomonas vaginalis and bacterial vaginosis)	1		1		1		1		2	2	2	2
	(d) Increased risk of STIs	1		1		1		1		2/3[b]	2	2/3[b]	2
Smoking	(a) Age <35	2		1		1		1		1		1	
	(b) Age ≥35, <15 cigarettes/day	3		1		1		1		1		1	
	(c) Age ≥35, >15 cigarettes/day	4		1		1		1		1		1	
Solid organ transplantation[a]	(a) Complicated	4		2		2		2		3	2	3	2
	(b) Uncomplicated	2[b]		2		2		2		2		2	

Stroke[a]	History of cerebrovascular accident	4	2	3	3	2	3	2	1
Superficial venous thrombosis	(a) Varicose veins	1	1	1	1	1	1	1	1
	(b) Superficial thrombophlebitis	2	1	1	1	1	1	1	1
Systemic lupus erythematosus[a]	(a) Positive (or unknown) antiphospholipid antibodies	4	3	3	3	3	3	3	1
	(b) Severe thrombocytopenia	2	2	3	2	2	2	3	2
	(c) Immunosuppressive treatment	2	2	2	2	2	2	2	1
	(d) None of the above	2	2	2	2	2	2	1	1
Thrombogenic mutations[a]		4[b]	2[b]	2[b]	2[b]	2[b]	2[b]	2[b]	1[b]
Thyroid disorders	Simple goiter/hyperthyroid/hypothyroid	1	1	1	1	1	1	1	
Tuberculosis[a] (see also drug interactions)	(a) Non-pelvic	1[b]	1[b]	1[b]	1[b]	1[b]	1[b]	1	
	(b) Pelvic	1[b]	1[b]	1[b]	1[b]	4	3	4	3
Unexplained vaginal bleeding	(Suspicious for serious condition) before evaluation	2[b]	2[b]	3[b]	3[b]	3[b]	4[b]	2[b]	4[b]	2[b]
Uterine fibroids		1	1	1	1	1	2	2	2

(continued)

(continued)

Condition	Sub-condition	Combined pill, patch, ring		Progestin-only pill		Injection		Implant		LNG-IUD		Copper-IUD	
		I	C	I	C	I	C	I	C	I	C	I	C
Valvular heart disease	(a) Uncomplicated	2		1		1		1		1		1	
	(b) Complicated[a]	4		1		1		1		1		1	
Vaginal bleeding patterns	(a) Irregular pattern without heavy bleeding	1		2		2		2		1	1	1	1
	(b) Heavy or prolonged bleeding	1[b]		2[b]		2[b]		2[b]		1[b]	2[b]	2[b]	2[b]
Viral hepatitis	(a) Acute or flare	3/4[b]	2	1		1		1		1		1	
	(b) Carrier/chronic	1	1	1		1		1		1		1	
Drug interactions													
Antiretroviral therapy	(a) Nucleoside reverse transcriptase inhibitors	1[b]		1		1		1		2/3[b]	2[b]	2/3[b]	2[b]
	(b) Non-nucleoside reverse transcriptase inhibitors	2[b]		2[b]		1		2[b]		2/3[b]	2[b]	2/3[b]	2[b]
	(c) Ritonavir-boosted protease inhibitors	3[b]		3[b]		1		2[b]		2/3[b]	2[b]	2/3[b]	2[b]

Anticonvulsant therapy	(a) Certain anticonvulsants (phenytoin, carbamazepine, barbiturates, primidone, topiramate, and oxcarbazepine)	3[b]	3[b]	1	3[b]	1	2[b]	1
	(b) Lamotrigine	3[b]	1	1	1	1	1	1
Antimicrobial therapy	(a) Broad spectrum antibiotics	1	1	1	1	1	1	1
	(b) Antifungals	1	1	1	1	1	1	1
	(c) Antiparasitics	1	1	1	1	1	1	1
	(d) Rifampicin or rifabutin therapy	3[b]	3[b]	1	2[b]	1	2[b]	1

AIDS acquired immunodeficiency syndrome, *BMI* body mass index, *C* continuation of contraceptive method, *COC* combined oral contraceptive, *Cu-IUD* copper-containing intrauterine device, *DVT* deep venous thrombosis, *hCG* human chorionic gonadotropin, *HIV* human immunodeficiency virus, *I* initiation of contraceptive method, *LNG-IUD* levonorgestrel-releasing intrauterine device, *NA* not applicable, *PE* pulmonary embolism, *STI* sexually transmitted infection, *VTE* venous thromboembolism

Source: Modified from CDC. Summary chart of US medical eligibility criteria for contraceptive use. Atlanta, GA: CDC; 2012 (available at http://www.cdc.gov/reproductivehealth/UnintendedPregnancy/USMEC. htm)

[a]Condition that exposes a woman to increased risk as a result of unintended pregnancy

[b]Please see the complete guidance for a clarification to this classification: www.cdc.gov/reproductivehealth/unintendedpregnancy/USMEC.htm

Appendix C
When to Start Using Specific Contraceptive Methods

Contraceptive method	When to start (if the provider is reasonably certain that the woman is not pregnant[a])	Additional contraception (i.e., backup) needed	Examinations or tests needed before initiation[b]
Copper-containing IUD	Anytime	Not needed	Bimanual examination and cervical inspection[c]
Levonorgestrel-releasing IUD	Anytime	If >7 days after menses started, use backup method or abstain for 7 days	Bimanual examination and cervical inspection[c]
Implant	Anytime	If >5 days after menses started, use backup method or abstain for 7 days	None

(continued)

A. Whitaker and M. Gilliam (eds.), *Contraception for Adolescent and Young Adult Women*, DOI 10.1007/978-1-4614-6579-9,

(continued)

Contraceptive method	When to start (if the provider is reasonably certain that the woman is not pregnant[a])	Additional contraception (i.e., backup) needed	Examinations or tests needed before initiation[b]
Injectable	Anytime	If >7 days after menses started, use backup method or abstain for 7 days	None
Combined hormonal contraceptive	Anytime	If >5 days after menses started, use backup method or abstain for 7 days	Blood pressure measurement
Progestin-only pill	Anytime	If >5 days after menses started, use backup method or abstain for 2 days	None

BMI body mass index, *HIV* human immunodeficiency virus, *IUD* intrauterine device, *STD* sexually transmitted disease, *US MEC US Medical Eligibility Criteria for Contraceptive Use, 2010*

Source: Centers for Disease Control and Prevention (CDC). U.S. Selected Practice Recommendations for Contraceptive Use, 2013. MMWR Recomm Rep. 2013;62(5):1–64.

[a]A provider can be reasonably sure that the woman is not pregnant when a woman has no signs or symptoms of pregnancy and meets any *one* of the following criteria: ≤7 days after start of normal menses, no intercourse since start of last normal menses, correct and consistent use of a reliable method of contraception, ≤7 days after spontaneous or induced abortion, within 4 weeks postpartum, or meet the criteria for lactational amenorrhea (fully or nearly fully breastfeeding, within 6 months postpartum, and amenorrheic)

(continued)

[b]Weight (BMI) measurement is not needed to determine medical eligibility for any methods of contraception because all methods can be used (US MEC 1) or generally can be used (US MEC 2) among obese women. However, measuring weight and calculating BMI (weight [kg]/height [m]^2) at baseline might be helpful for monitoring any changes and counseling women who might be concerned about weight change perceived to be associated with their contraceptive method

[c]Most women do not require additional STD screening at the time of IUD insertion if they have already been screened according to CDC's *STD Treatment Guidelines* (available at http://www.cdc.gov/std/treatment). If a woman has not been screened according to guidelines, screening can be performed at the time of IUD insertion, and insertion should not be delayed. Women with purulent cervicitis or current chlamydial infection or gonorrhea should not undergo IUD insertion (US MEC 4). Women who have a very high individual likelihood of STD exposure (e.g., those with a currently infected partner) generally should not undergo IUD insertion (US MEC 3). For these women, IUD insertion should be delayed until appropriate testing and treatment occurs

Index

A

Abortion
  and adoption, 210
  age, 205
  decision making, 206
  functions, counselor, 206
  mental health, 212
  methods, 206
  minor's decision, 210, 211
  network, 213
  postabortion, 213
  rate, 205, 206
  safety and outcomes, 211
  teen, 206
  US, 205, 206
Adolescents
  CHC (*see* Combined hormonal
    contraception (CHC))
  COCs, 5
  contraceptive care (*see*
    Contraception)
  coping/mental health, 212
  IUD (*see* Intrauterine device
    (IUD))
  legal and policy
    confidentiality (*see*
      Confidentiality and
      contraceptive care)
    framework, 193
    minor consent (*see* Minor
      consent laws)

obese (*see* Obese)
  POCs (*see* Progestin-only
    contraception (POCs))
  postpartum (*see* Postpartum
    contraception)
  sexuality education (*see*
    Sexuality)
  side effects (*see* Side effects)
Adolescent sexual and
    reproductive health
    (ASRH), 179–180
Adoption and prenatal care
  abortion, 208
  agency and private, 207
  counseling session, 209
  definition, 207
  financial/emotional support,
    209
  functions, counselor's, 209
  knowledge, pregnancy, 209
  pregnancy options
    workbook, 208
Antiepileptic drugs (AEDs), 156
ASRH. *See* Adolescent sexual
    and reproductive
    health (ASRH)
Asthma
  contraceptive methods and
    cautions, 124–125
  control, 124
  prevalence, 124

A. Whitaker and M. Gilliam (eds.), *Contraception for Adolescent
and Young Adult Women*, DOI 10.1007/978-1-4614-6579-9,
© Springer Science + Business Media New York 2014

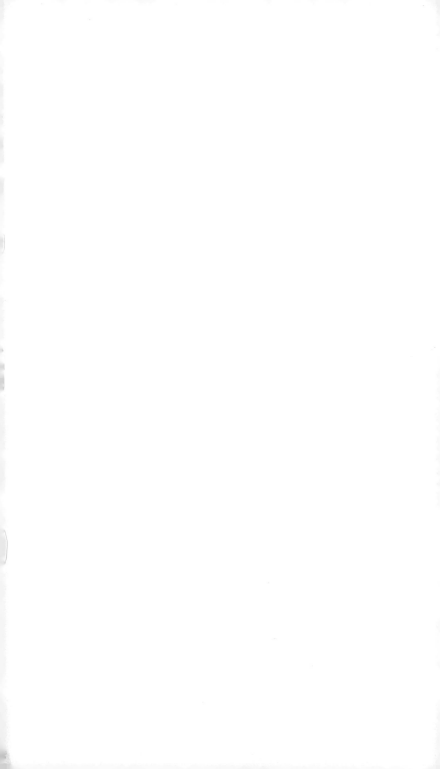

Printed by Publishers' Graphics LLC
DBT140722.23.35.1